STABILITY WORKOUTS ON THE
BALANCE BOARD

STABILITY WORKOUTS <small>ON THE</small>
BALANCE BOARD

Illustrated Step-by-Step Guide to Toning, Strengthening and Rehabilitative Techniques

Dr. Karl Knopf

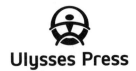

Ulysses Press

Published in the United States by:
Ulysses Press
P.O. Box 3440
Berkeley, CA 94703
www.ulyssespress.com

ISBN: 978-1-61243-490-2
Library of Congress Control Number: 2015937562

Printed in the United States by Bang Printing
10 9 8 7 6 5 4 3 2 1

Acquisitions: Kelly Reed
Managing editor: Claire Chun
Editor: Lily Chou
Proofreader: Nancy Bell
Indexer: Sayre Van Young
Front cover/interior design and layout: what!design @ whatweb.com
Cover artwork: people © Rapt Productions, studio © fiphoto/shutterstock.com, starburst © FMStox/shutterstock.com
Interior artwork: Rapt Productions except page 2 © Margaret Knopf, page 3 © Anatoli Styf/shutterstock.com, page 121 © Margaret Knopf
Models: Nadia Brunner-Velasquez, Christopher Wells, Bryan Ausinheiler (front cover), Caitlin Halferty (front cover)
Make-Up: SabrinaFosterMakeup.com

Distributed by Publishers Group West

CONTENTS

PART 1
OVERVIEW
1

PART 2
PROGRAMS
19

PART 3
EXERCISES
31

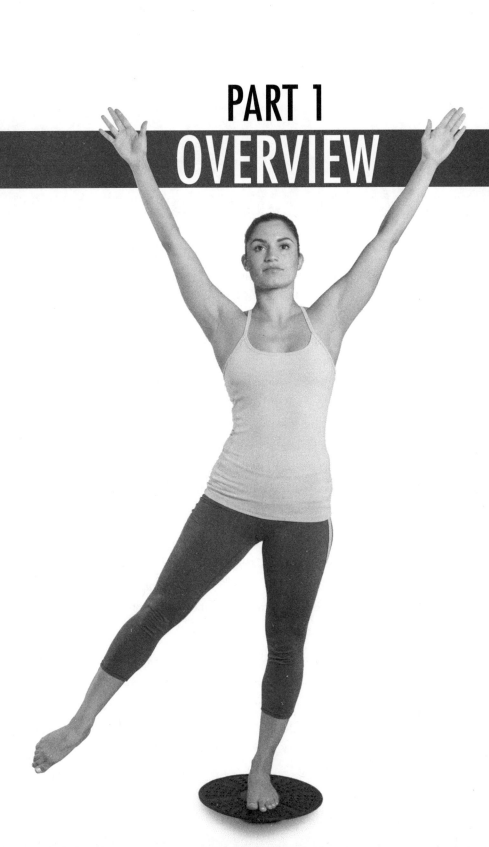

PART 1
OVERVIEW

BUILDING BETTER BALANCE WITH A BALANCE BOARD

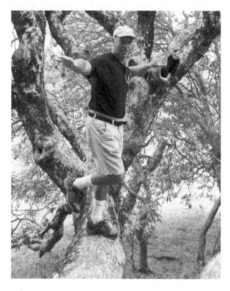

Do you want a full and fun life? If yes, then having good balance is the answer! Everything we do, from riding a horse to paddleboarding to window shopping with our friends, entails having adequate balance. Good balance is more than standing on one leg, though. It can, among many other things, also involve sitting upright, unsupported, and walking across the wet stones of a creek. Functional balance is critical for everyone, from tightrope walkers to wounded warriors trying to regain their ability to walk again. The loss of functional balance could inhibit even the simplest activities of daily living, from climbing a ladder to curtailing our involvement in sports that we love. Poor balance often leads to falls, which account for a large number of visits to the emergency room.

When we're young and lose our balance, we often laugh it off since the only damage done is to our ego. As we get older, however, a simple fall can contribute to serious injury, whether it's a fractured wrist, dislocated shoulder or, worse yet, a broken hip. It can't be understated that appropriate balance is a critical component of everyday living, from maintaining balance on the athletic field to simply being able to navigate around the house.

Start now to maintain or regain your balance. The balance board is an effective tool for targeting both the superficial and deep-lying muscles of the body that affect balance. Operating on the idea that muscular control is one of the keys to good functional balance, *Stability Workouts on the Balance Board* offers safe, straightforward exercises that strengthen all muscles, both major and minor, engaged in balance. Whether you're rehabbing from an injury or waking up early every morning to surf the waves, you'll benefit from these balance-board movements.

WHAT IS BALANCE?

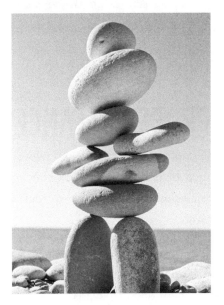

Balance is defined as "the ability to maintain the center of a mass over the base of support." This is evident even when you see rocks strategically stacked on top of each other to produce sculptures. Human balance, however, is more problematic than setting rocks on top of each other because we must keep our equilibrium under a variety of disturbances, such as walking on uneven terrain, running or maintaining balance on a moving train. Graceful balance is critical to quality of life and is the result of maintaining equilibrium in both posture and alignment, whether you're standing still on a balance bar or moving smoothly across a gymnastics floor.

There are two types of balance: static balance and dynamic balance.

Static balance involves remaining stationary in one place for a period of time. Examples of static balance include standing on one or even two legs without moving or maintaining solid balance on our hands and knees without shaking.

Dynamic balance is being able to move effortlessly and gracefully from one place to the next at any given speed, or to be able to change direction quickly while still maintaining balance. It's said that "walking is basically falling forward from one step to the next." That, of course, is an oversimplification because walking requires concentric contractions of certain muscles to propel us forward and eccentric contractions to decelerate us from falling forward. In other words, asking the body to move from one spot to the next while still maintaining a balanced posture involves a complex sequence of neuromuscular interactions. Walking, full-body turns, and quick "cuts" in sports, jumping and landing are all examples of dynamic balance.

Some mobility experts consider walking as falling forward yet catching ourselves before we fall completely to the ground. You might say, "I don't fall," but fall-prevention experts deem that "tripping" but catching yourself is technically a fall. The more often we "trip," the greater the risk the next one will be.

To maintain good balance, our body needs to know when to engage certain muscles while relaxing others. Even overreaching for an object can throw us off balance, while a quick turn of the head can cause us to stumble. Some people even find that moving from sitting to standing can cause them to lose their balance. However, we often improve our balance without consciously knowing it, such as when we automatically lower our center of gravity when walking across a slippery surface or see that we're going to be bumped. We also know that if our shoes have traction, the better our balance will be on wet surfaces.

SENSORY ELEMENTS NEEDED FOR PROPER BALANCE

Too many people think that just practicing standing on one leg will improve their balance. However, improving balance is no simple task! Maintaining or developing good balance is a complex concept that involves many concomitant issues such as good posture, which can include anticipatory and reactive postural control (i.e., being able to adjust quickly to different situations).

Balance can be influenced by medical conditions (such as a stroke or Parkinson's disease), visual impairments, medications, or even the results of damage caused to the peripheral sensory systems by diabetes. For most people, though, balance is affected by how we see, hear and feel things.

Visual. When the sensory receptors of the eye are stimulated, they send messages through the optic nerve to the balance center of the brain (brainstem). These messages include information about our surroundings. In the simplest terms, the eyes "see" the surroundings and send a message to the brain. The brainstem then deciphers and relays information to the motor fibers that carry impulses to the muscles of the eyes and the muscles that need to contract or relax to adjust to the stimuli. Unfortunately, eye conditions such as macular degeneration, glaucoma and cataracts can contribute to the "eyes" not seeing the stimuli properly.

Vestibular. The sensory receptors of the vestibular system located in the inner ear provide information about head movement and position. When we move our head, the fluid within the semicircular canals of the inner ear sends signals via the vestibular nerves to the balance center of the brain. The vestibular system is a major player in maintaining balance. Remember spinning around quickly as a kid and then trying to walk straight? It was a fun game as a kid, but if it happened every day it would be devastating (ask anyone who's ever had a bout of vertigo).

Somatosensitive or Proprioceptive. The somatosensory system is responsible for our ability to maintain postural control. The sensory receptors in our muscles and joints are stimulated by touch, pressure and movement. Proprioception is the system that interprets the information sent back and forth to the brain about the surface you're on, what you're touching, and the position of your body. There are two parts of the feedback loop: One sends messages up the spinal cord to the brain; the brain then processes the information and sends it back down the spinal cord to the muscle/joint, telling it how to react. This all happens in a matter of microseconds. Proprioception provides the information needed to perform coordinated movements. However, a defect anywhere in the system (for instance, a brain injury) can impair balance.

OTHER FACTORS THAT INFLUENCE BALANCE

Many variables can influence our ability to maintain ideal balance.

Chronic conditions. Many common chronic conditions, including arthritis, diabetes and neurological issues, influence a person's ability to maintain proper balance. Unfortunately, sometimes a chronic condition leads to poor posture and weak muscles as a result of disuse. If a person has a significant disability, it's imperative that he do as much as possible to maintain a functional level of balance to perform activities of daily living. No amount of balance training, however, will help to improve balance if there's a defect in the systems. The more limiting the condition, the more important it is that a trained personnel oversee the balance-training program. Sad fact: Arthritis is the number-one cause of disability in America. It's often quoted that what sends someone to a nursing home is not a person's age or disability but rather their ability to ambulate and care for themselves. The fear of falling is a major concern for older individuals, which often makes them housebound.

Age. No matter how well we've maintained ourselves, age-related changes could lead to balance limitations. While age alone doesn't cause balance problems, some of the changes seen in aging can influence a person's balance. Fortunately, age-related changes might not occur in every individual. The great unknown is why some people manifest limitations as they get older while others never display any loss of function.

Medications/drugs. Many medications and drugs interfere with balance. Whether it's prescribed or an over-the-counter medication, it can still have a deleterious effect upon a person's balance and coordination. Some medications contribute to postural hypotension that leads to fainting, dizziness and weakness. Often, the more medications (four or more) a person is on, the greater the influence they have. Also, it has been found that older clients (65 years and over) can't tolerate medications the same way younger folks can. In addition, it goes without saying that medication combined with alcohol, marijuana and other recreational drugs can only compound the effects upon balance and coordination.

Anyone with balance dysfunctions should consult a physician and their pharmacist regarding the interaction of their medications. Always read the side-effects insert that accompanies your medications. It's also wise to have a gatekeeper, whether it's your primary-care physician or using just one pharmacy, to oversee all your medications.

Proper hydration. As silly as this may sound, inadequate hydration can play a role in balance. Some people may not hydrate themselves enough because of bladder concerns. Older people and athletes often don't recognize that they're not properly hydrated, which can play a part in experiencing postural hypotension/fainting.

Some common things to watch out for:

- If you're thirsty, you're already dehydrated.

- The darker your urine is, the less hydrated you are. Aim for at least one lighter-colored urine a day.

- Some medications cause you to lose fluids.

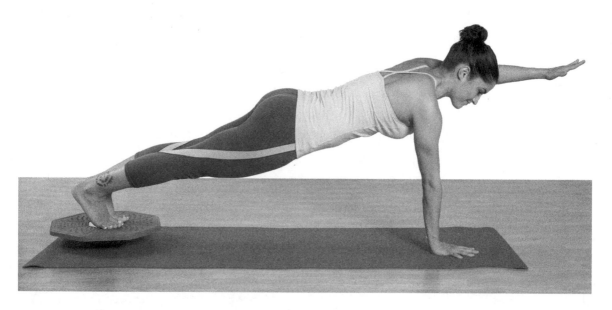

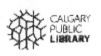

CALGARY
PUBLIC
LIBRARY

Quarry Park
Self Checkout
February,15,2019 09:53

39065147426660   3/8/2019
Stability workouts on the balance board
 : illustrated step-by-step guide to to
ning, strengthening and rehabilitative
techniques

Total   **1 item(s)**

You have 0 item(s) ready for pickup

THE ANATOMY OF BALANCE

As the old song goes, the ankle bone is connected to the knee bone, which is connected to the hip bone, which is connected to the torso and to the neck. But without a brain and an intact neurological system to send messages up and down the spine, nothing would happen. Without a sufficient muscular system, nothing would move.

For starters, the ankle joint and the supporting muscles of the ankle and lower leg play a significant role in maintaining balance. Limited ankle flexibility, in fact, can impair balance. The toes are also valuable players when it comes to balance.

The hip joint is the powerhouse joint of the lower body, and the muscles of the hip joint are much stronger than the muscles of the ankle. Hip-joint mobility and strength allow for forward and backward movement of the leg. The pelvic area serves as a base of support for the upper extremities. Together, the hip and ankle joints are critical for functional balance. Even the simple task of walking would be very difficult without the integrated function of these two joints.

The torso is the platform that the head relies on for proper positioning. The core is made up of many layers of muscles, including the abdominal muscles at the front, the obliques at the sides, and the erector spinae group at the back. If any of these are imbalanced, you'll have a difficult time standing erect. Think of a weak core as a wet noodle.

WHY IS BALANCE IMPORTANT?

Most people understand the importance of strength training and aerobic exercise, and some remember to do flexibility work, but often we never find time to include balance work in our session. Proper balance is critical to an active and engaged lifestyle. Good functional balance allows us to maintain balance, whether standing on an unstable surface (such as a balance board), standing on one leg (single support) while reaching for an object, or standing on two legs (dual support) during a bumpy bus ride. Even sitting upright requires some level of torso balance.

The changes in balance are often so gradual that we don't notice them until we have major issues. The concept of functional balance seems effortless yet is very complex and requires all systems to be working well together. When our balance system is off, we run the risk of falling or tripping. Worse yet, a fear of falling can limit our joy of living.

ASSESSMENT

While many trainers use standing on one leg to evaluate balance, this type of assessment only measures static balance and doesn't always translate into functional balance. In real life we need to be able to sit and stand as well as ambulate without looking awkward.

The following simple assessment is a quick intuitive tool to see how you feel while doing it. Don't perform it if you have questionable balance. It's recommended that you use this tool in a pre- and post-test format: Evaluate yourself now and then every three months after doing balance work regularly. Keep in mind that you're not competing with anyone—all that's important is that you continue progressing.

1. Stand with both feet together and your eyes open. Now close them. Did you notice a difference between having your eyes closed and having them open? (Vision plays a significant role in balance.)

2. Sit in a chair with the chair securely pressed up against a wall. Time how quickly you can walk out 10 feet, turn around, return to the chair, and sit down.

3. Walk quickly from point A to point B and have someone tell you to stop quickly. Could you stop quickly? Did you overshoot your spot?

4. Walk 10 feet very slowly, heel to toe. (Most people with balance issues find that walking very slowly is harder than walking quickly.)

Is your balance as good as you expected? If so, great! If not, start out slowly and safely, performing the basic balance moves starting on page 14 first and then progressing to the exercises in Part 3 as you improve.

These simple functional tests are aimed at involving real life situations and to see how you respond in a controlled environment. Track your results over the next few months and see if you improve.

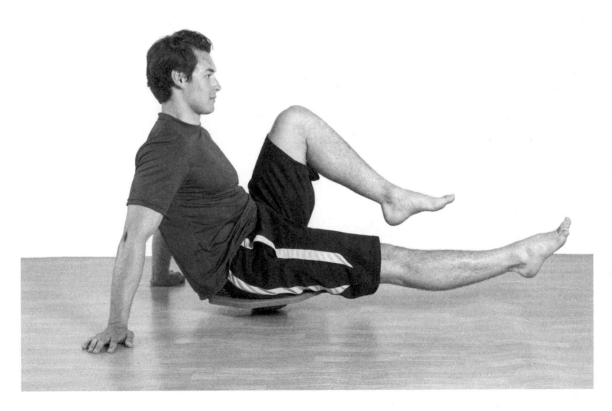

WHAT IS A BALANCE BOARD?

While balance exercises on the ground are useful and productive and should always be the port of entry for balance training, it's critical to challenge your balance systems as you progress. This is where the balance board comes in. Balance boards come in a variety of shapes and sizes but, conceptually, they all work the same way. Whether they're a wobble board, rocker, foam pad or inflatable disk, they all ask the user to maintain balance while on an unstable surface.

Balance boards engage both the superficial and deep-lying muscles of the body that affect balance. Since they come in different shapes and sizes, the type of board you choose should match your skill set and desired goal. Some people see the balance board as a simple toy while others view it as exercise equipment or even a therapeutic device.

The great thing about balance boards is that they're an inexpensive, effective and portable exercise tool for challenging the complex systems that influence balance. These simple devices can increase core strength, improve balance, tone muscles and rehabilitate injuries—all of which can be done either at home or at the gym. The role that the balance board plays is determined by the goal intended by the user. A child steps on it and finds it fun to see how long she can stay on it. The fitness enthusiast experiments with it while exercising. In the hands of a health professional, it's a tool to improve functional mobility and ambulation in someone with balance dysfunction.

Standing on the balance board can present the potential for a fall so it's wise to place the device on a sticky exercise mat or rough carpet so that the board doesn't slip out from under you. Also make sure that the area around you is free of hazardous objects.

BEFORE YOU BEGIN

Before participating in a balance-board routine, take a truthful assessment of your balance skill set. Can you stand on one foot with and without your eyes open? Can you walk in and out of a crowded store without bumping into people? While you may be in good shape with regard to cardiovascular fitness or physical strength, you may not be as good with balance as you think. Consider taking a few moments to take the balance-evaluation assessment on page 8. If you have a preexisting condition, such as a visual concern or a neurological consideration, it's wise to consult your health professional before trying any of the exercises in this book.

When starting a balance-training program, forget the old paradigm of reps and sets. Balance training is not about reps and sets—it's very much a total mind/body experience. For instance, one day you may be able to hold a position but the next day, when you're preoccupied or fatigued, you may find that you're unsteady.

Near my beach house is a railroad track. Every time I walk my dogs down the path, I see how far I can walk on the rails before falling off. I never go the same distance—if I get distracted, I fall off quickly; if I can keep my mind on the task at hand, I can go pretty far. Your balance-training progress will inevitably vary from day to day, but don't get frustrated! Remember: For best results, be in the moment. To gain the most from these balance-board exercises, do them when you have the time to focus on what you're doing.

You'll quickly notice that balance training is similar to downhill skiing or hitting a golf ball—sometimes you just find the "groove," and then the next time you feel completely uncoordinated. My hope is that the more you practice balance-board training, the more positive experiences you'll have.

FAQS

Here are some common questions about balance-board training.

Q. When should I engage in balance training?

A. For best results, balance training should be performed when you're fresh and in a quiet place void of distractions.

Q. Should I do a preset program first?

A. Some people like chocolate ice cream, some like vanilla—neither one is right or wrong. So it is with a balance-board program. If you like structure, then select a predetermined program until you feel comfortable being creative. If you know your body and its abilities and limitations, try making up a routine. Some days it might be easier to perform a preset program and add a few sprinkles on your program for flair.

Q. How do I select exercises?

A. The exercises/activities in Part 3 are organized by position. The ones listed first in each section are generally the most basic; their difficulty level progresses to more challenging. I've provided some preset programs in Part 2 to make it easier to get started. However, if you're like me and don't like to be told what to do, you can pick and choose movements and see how they resonate with your mood, skill set and performance. Each of us has special balance abilities, so what might be easy for you might be difficult for someone else. A little sampling and experimentation is the best way to go when creating the best balance program for your needs.

FIT TIP: No matter what your skill level is, it's recommended that you begin at the basic level.

If you have good balance, you'll progress through each level quickly until you reach a level that challenges you.

Q. How often should you train?

A. Unlike power training that requires a "rest" period to recover, balance activities can be performed daily and maybe even several times a day. The key to improving balance is to perform them when you have time and intention to focus on them. Just "plugging" them into an existing program because someone told you you "should" is of no productive use. Never let anyone "should" you!

Q. Do I need to warm up for these exercises?

A. You really don't need a formal warm-up to participate in balance-board movements. However, if you're stiff and have aching joints, it would be well advised to participate in your balance-board activities when you're at your optimum with regard to mind and body. So if you feel like you could use a warm-up, feel free to do so.

Q. Should I wear shoes or go barefoot?

A. The correct answer: Do whatever provides you with enough friction to "grip" plus feel the board. Believe it or not, allowing your toes to feel the board can impact your balance. When I worked in an amputee ward at the VA hospital, I learned that patients who had the benefit of their big toe had much better balance than those who had lost their toes to diabetes.

Q. You say the exercises should "feel right" but what does that mean?

A. "Feels right" means it's time to listen to your body. In today's society, people are always "plugged in"—they watch TV while they run on the treadmill, listen to music while lifting weights, check their Fitbit to see if their workout was acceptable. What can your body tell you about the exercise? Did you feel uncomfortable while doing it? Did you feel awkward while performing the move? Were you shaky or rock steady when you were holding a pose? As a very old healer once said, "Listen to your body and it will tell you the cure!" If you're always looking for objective measures about your performance, you might be missing some important messages.

SOME TIPS WHEN USING THE BALANCE BOARD

- The single-leg standing series are best done while standing barefoot in the center of board.

- Generally these boards are hard and sitting on them may get uncomfortable; don't do prolonged sitting. Get up after each exercise and move around. You might also place a pad or cushion on top of the board for comfort.

- All of the stretches done on the balance board are considered advanced. If you're not ready to perform them on a balance board, you'll receive the same flexibility benefit by doing the stretch while just standing on the floor.

GETTING STARTED ON THE BALANCE BOARD

Everyone should start here. Don't skip this section, even if you're an elite gymnastics star. If you have super balance, you'll progress through this section quickly and easily. This section can also be used as a personal assessment section—you might be surprised how some of these very basic moves can be very challenging.

Do not stand on the board until you've mastered these exercises. Do not progress to the exercises in Part 3 until you can do *all* of these moves without assistance or support. Once you've graduated to using a balance board, the goal and expectation of the balance-board exercises is to progress to the point where you can perform them without the use of any external support. However, while you're attempting to improve your balance-board skill, you may use a chair, wall or partner as necessary.

STANDING STARTER WITHOUT BOARD

TARGET: Core, leg stamina

1 Stand near a chair with your feet a comfortable distance apart and weight evenly supported by both feet. Hold on to the back of the chair if needed.

2 Close your eyes. See how long you can maintain your balance; without holding on to the chair, 30 seconds or more would be ideal. Note how much you sway.

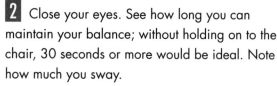

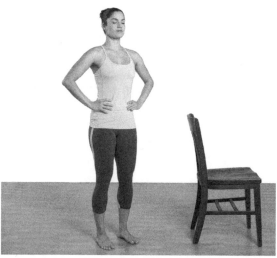

SINGLE-LEG STANDING STARTER WITHOUT BOARD

TARGET: Core, leg stamina

1 Stand near a chair with your feet a comfortable distance apart and weight evenly supported by both feet. Hold on to the back of the chair if needed.

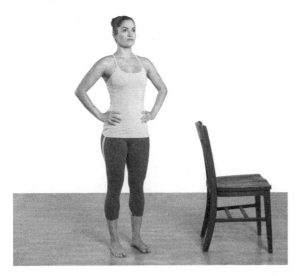

2 Lift your weaker leg off the floor a few inches. See how long you can maintain your balance; without holding on to the chair, 30 seconds or more would be ideal. Note how much you sway.

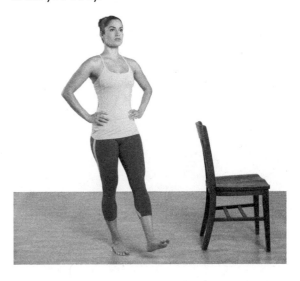

Try the same movement with the other leg. Do you notice a difference between legs?

ADVANCED VARIATION: Try this with your eyes closed.

SINGLE-LEG STANDING HEAD TURN WITHOUT BOARD

TARGET: Core, leg stamina

1 Stand near a chair with your feet a comfortable distance apart and weight evenly supported by both feet. Hold on to the back of the chair if needed.

2 Lift your weaker leg off the floor a few inches and slowly look to the left. Hold the pose for a few seconds.

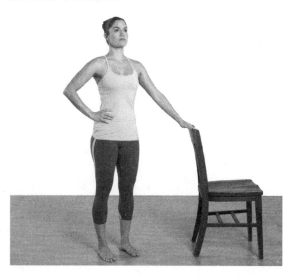

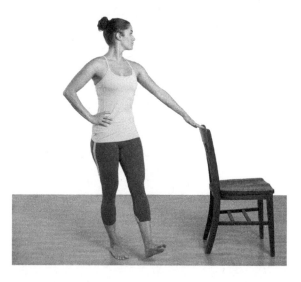

Return to start position and repeat on the other side.

ADVANCED VARIATION: Try this with your eyes closed.

FORWARD LEAN WITHOUT BOARD

TARGET: Leg stamina

1 Stand an arm's distance from a wall or solid chair, with your feet a comfortable distance apart and weight evenly supported by both feet.

2 Lean slightly forward as far as possible while maintaining balance. Try not to use the support.

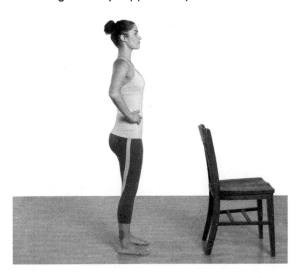

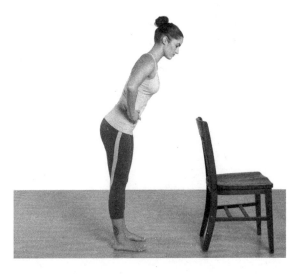

Return to start position.

ADVANCED VARIATION: Try doing this move to both sides as well as back and forth.

BICYCLE PEDAL WITHOUT BOARD

TARGET: Core, leg stamina

Try to use only minimal help from the chair, progressing from a grip to a fingertip touch to no touching.

1 Stand an arm's distance from a wall or solid chair, with your feet a comfortable distance apart and weight evenly supported by both feet.

2–3 While maintaining balance, lift your weaker leg off the floor a few inches and pedal forward as if you're pedaling a bike.

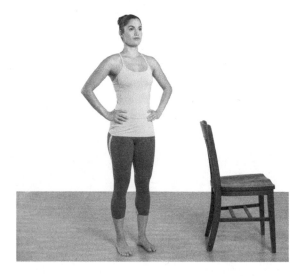

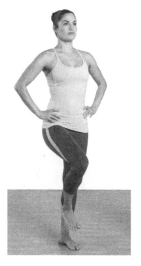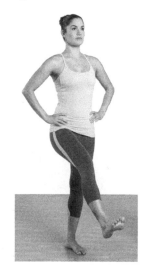

Return to start position and lift the other leg and perform the same motion.

Return to start position and repeat on the other side.

ADVANCED VARIATION: Try this with your eyes closed.

PART 2
PROGRAMS

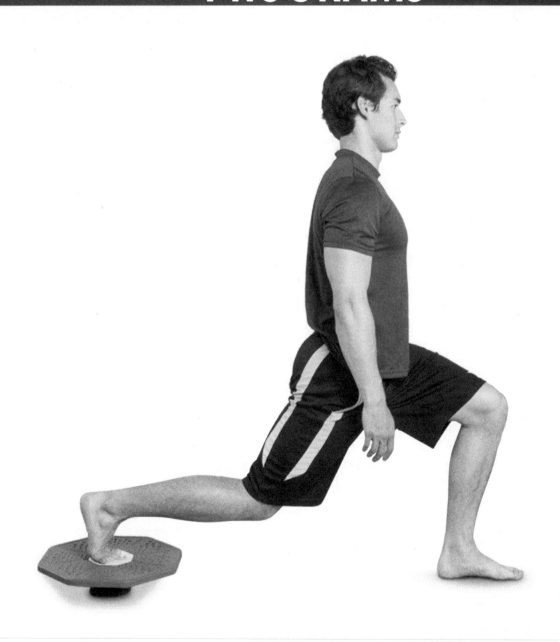

HOW TO USE THIS BOOK

The aim of this book is to offer something for everyone, from folks trying to regain their balance after an injury to athletes who do stunts their mothers told them never to do. Safety should always be your number-one priority. You're the captain of your body and no one knows you better than you. Don't let anyone "should" you!

Prior to starting any of the balance-board programs or exercises, please take a moment and perform the assessment (page 8). This will give you a rudimentary understanding of your balance proficiency. After taking the assessment, allow yourself time to do an introspective appraisal of your abilities as well as consider what your goals may be. The destination of balance has many routes—select the route that gives you joy and satisfaction. We as humans tend to repeat those activities that bring us pleasure.

Once you have figured out your abilities by performing the assessment and then deciding on a goal, you may choose a pre-designed program (starting on page 23) or pick exercises from Part 3 that you feel will best serve your needs. While specific target areas are mentioned for each exercise, all of these exercises work on proprioception, body awareness, understanding how to adjust your body-weight distribution, and learning how to compensate for your center of gravity as you move around—all of which are crucial for improving overall balance.

Safety first! It's always wise to place the balance board on a sticky exercise mat or rough carpet so that the board doesn't slip out from under you. Also make sure that the area around you is free of hazardous objects in case you fall.

HOW SHOULD I TRACK MY TRAINING?

Since reps and sets are not the best method to address balance training, time is the best indicator of improvement. Use a large clock with a second hand to time your position or use an app on your phone. It's best to start wherever you're at, so if all you can do is hold the position for 1 second, then your goal is to improve to 5 seconds. Continue aiming to add 5 seconds to your hold time until you reach 30 seconds or even 1 minute. Keep in mind, however, that 60 seconds of wiggling all about is *not* better than 30 seconds of steady posture. You're ready for the next exercise when you can hold a stable position steadily for 30 seconds or more.

Training with a friend is a great option. They can not only time you but spot you for safety and provide feedback. Performing the moves in front of a mirror or even using your phone to record your movement is a great way to see how you're doing.

If none of the above are viable options, consider using your internal monitoring system and asking yourself:

- How did you feel?

- Did you feel more or less steady?

- Were your legs or torso struggling to maintain balance?

It's fine to repeat the activity as many times as you wish. Balance training is not about hard and fast rules. Enjoy the process.

CREATING YOUR OWN ROUTINE

You know yourself best. Therefore, by designing your own program, you're selecting exercises based on your ability and motivation level. Your balance program should be a living document that changes regularly as you advance or regress. You might also have seasonal programs that match your recreational interests, such as a ski program for the winter and surfing program for the summer.

After you've participated in the balance assessment (page 8), you should have a basic understanding of your skill set. For example, you have excellent static balance but you've discovered that your dynamic balance is questionable. Or you may notice that when you dart quickly in and around people in a crowded area you often falter. So take time to reflect what you do best and which areas you notice deficits and then select exercises that focus on a particular area.

Your routine doesn't have to be set in stone! As you change, adapt your program to your current skill level. In fact, consider changing your program regularly. If you don't modify the program periodically, you'll probably plateau and not progress (not to mention get very bored and quit).

Remember: Any exercise program meant to improve balance should not only teach balance skills but also include a foundation of related flexibility and strength activities. Strength and stamina help us control our center of mass, and muscular strength and proper flexibility are fundamental to balance training.

10 BALANCE-TRAINING TIPS

1. Work toward symmetrical developmental of the muscular system (meaning work your front side as much as your back side, from your ankles to your torso). A misaligned posture, such as a forward head or rounded shoulders, can throw your balance off. Make sure to not overstrengthen one set of muscles.

2. Maintain adequate hip strength and flexibility ratios, primarily in the gluteal muscles and hamstrings as well as the quadriceps.

3. Focus on the muscles of the core and lower extremities.

4. Perform static moves before progressing to active ones.

5. Perform easy moves before difficult ones.

6. Whenever possible, try to perform movements that replicate activities of daily living (often called functional exercises).

7. Select moves that best prepare you for the goal you've determined. For instance, if you have a history of falling in line at the grocery store, select static moves that should be done to develop a solid platform to progress. Then select exercises similar to movements you perform at the store.

8. Always strive to perform movements with proper posture and head placement.

9. If you suspect a deficiency in your sensory, visual or neurological systems, seek medical attention. No amount of balance training will help if any of the systems are broken.

10. Never perform movements that are beyond what you can do safely.

BASIC PROGRAM (FOUNDATIONAL BALANCE)

This program is designed for improving functional balance in activities of daily living. Foundational balance activities should begin without the balance board and should focus on weight shifts and dual- and single-leg holds before graduating to basic through advanced moves on the balance board. As the old proverb states, "The journey of a thousand miles begin with a single step." So it is with balance—it's not where you start but where you end.

You don't have to do every exercise in this program. Listen to your body and it will tell you how many to do and how long to hold a position. Learn to be your own personal trainer!

EXERCISES

Seated Orientation,* page 32

Seated Leg Extension, page 35

Seated Chest Press, page 42

Seated Fly, page 44

Mad Cat, page 46

Pelvic Lift, page 58

Three-Point Sequence, page 48

Standing Starter, page 66

Standing Empire State Building,** page 71

Rock around the Clock, page 69

*Don't progress to any other exercises until you master this one.

**Don't progress to other standing exercises until you're safe with this exercise.

INTERMEDIATE PROGRAM

This program is designed for recreational athletes who find they trip a little more than usual and feel a little shaky when up on a ladder. Most of us are at this level.

You don't have to do every exercise in this program. Listen to your body and it will tell you how many to do and how long to hold a position. Learn to be your own personal trainer!

EXERCISES

Seated Frontal Raise, page 36

Seated Straight-Leg Raise, page 34

Seated Lateral Raise, page 37

Seated Horizontal Triceps Extension, page 40

Seated Chest Press, page 42

Mad Cat, page 46

Plank to Pike, page 50

Push-Up, page 54

Three-Point Sequence, page 48

Standing Starter,* page 66

Standing Forward Lean, page 67

Standing Empire State Building, page 71

Rock around the Clock, page 69

Forward Lunge, page 75

*Don't progress to other exercises until you're safe with this exercise.

ADVANCED PROGRAM

This program is for those who are like cats: They never trip and could walk a balance beam with their eyes closed. Once you feel ready, you can also try a couple of these exercises to challenge yourself. However, do not put yourself in harm's way. BE SAFE!

You don't have to do every exercise in this program. Listen to your body and it will tell you how many to do and how long to hold a position. Learn to be your own personal trainer!

EXERCISES

Standing Starter,* page 66

Rock Around the Clock, page 69

Dynamic Squat, page 78

Forward Lunge, page 75

Standing Lateral Arm Swing, page 80

Stork Stand, page 88

T Stand, page 91

Can Can Kick, page 60

Single-Leg Curl, page 94

Opposite Jacks, page 92

Single-Leg Extension, page 95

Lateral Single-Leg Raise, page 97

Single-Leg Stand with Torso Rotation, page 89

Chair Push-Up, page 68

Diamond Push-Up with Band, page 55

Side Plank, page 56

Standing Lateral Raise, page 81

Standing Row, page 86

Standing Overhead Press, page 87

Half Squat, page 72

*Don't progress to other exercises until you're safe with this exercise.

LAND SPORTS PROGRAM

Everyone marvels at the grace of a gymnast—they display both dynamic and static balance during every routine. If you've ever watched the X Games, you soon realize that skateboarding today is not as simple as what Jan and Dean sang about in their sidewalk surfing song. Another display of great balance and coordination is when people do stunts on bikes.

While doing the exercises in this book will not promise great levels of balance seen by these exceptional athletes, regular participation in a balance program can improve your functional balance. The moves included in this program will benefit you whether you're a softball, basketball or soccer player. Almost every sport we play requires some level of balance, so improved balance should help no matter what you play.

- If you have great balance and wish to invent a balance-board exercise specific to your sport, go for it!

- If you're a basketball player, try dribbling or passing the ball while on the board.

- If you're baseball player, try to play catch with a pal while on the board.

- If you're a gamer, try playing video games while standing on the board.

- If you're a talker, try talking on your cell phone while on the board.

Please note that most of the exercises in this section are rather challenging and it's completely acceptable to exchange these exercises for others that best meet your skill set. You're not required to perform all the movements in this routine. As always, listen to your body and it will tell you how much to do. Be your own best personal trainer and train safely.

EXERCISES

WATER SPORTS PROGRAM

Whether you're a surfer, waterskier, stand-up paddleboarder or kayaker, having good balance is an integral part of the enjoyment of the sport. To be a functional surfer, you must have the agility to stand up once you catch a wave and then be able to position your feet so that you can maintain your center of gravity as you maneuver the waves. A waterskier, while being pulled over an unpredictable surface at various speeds, has a similar challenge whether using double or single skis. The stand-up paddleboarder must be able to juggle her balance while paddling in a particular direction and also be able to adjust to the water's dynamic influences. Kayakers need good-seated balance and the ability to paddle while navigating boulders or waves.

Note that you don't have to do every exercise in this program. Listen to your body and it will tell you how many to do and how long to hold a position. Learn to be your own personal trainer!

You know your particular skill set in your sport; adapt the program as you deem appropriate.

EXERCISES	SPORT
Seated Reverse Fly, page 39	Kayaking
Seated Horizontal Triceps Extension (single or dual arms), page 40	Kayaking
Seated Row, page 41	Kayaking
Three-Point Sequence, page 48	All
Plank to Pike, page 50	All
Plank, page 51	All
Standing Forward Lean, page 67	Stand-up paddleboarding/Waterskiing
Opposite Jacks, page 92	Surfing/Stand-up paddleboarding/ Waterskiing
Rock around the Clock, page 69	Stand-up paddleboarding
Half Squat, page 72	All

SNOW SPORTS PROGRAM

Downhill skiing can be a lot of fun if you spend most of the day upright, but it can be a miserable sport if, during the majority of the day, you're in a faceplant position. Looking graceful and not falling can be difficult when you're asked to wax down your skis and slide over an icy surface, or while dodging mogul mice and then stopping gracefully at the end of the run. Balance, of course, is also at the core of cross-country skiing. Even though skiing is done in the winter, this program should be done year-round, not just as the snow falls.

Note that you don't have to do every exercise in this program. Listen to your body and it will tell you how many to do and how long to hold a position. Learn to be your own personal trainer!

You know your particular skill set in your sport; adapt the program as you deem appropriate.

EXERCISES	SPORT
Standing Forward Lean, page 67	Downhill and cross-country skiing
Half Squat (advanced variation), page 72	Downhill skiing
Side Step, page 77	Cross-country skiing
Standing Arm Swing, page 79	Downhill and cross-country skiing
Standing Frontal Raise (variation), page 82	Downhill and cross-country skiing
Forward Toe Tap, page 73	Downhill and cross-country skiing
Lateral Toe Tap, page 74	Downhill and cross-country skiing
Standing Horizontal Triceps Extension, page 84	Downhill and cross-country skiing

PART 3
EXERCISES

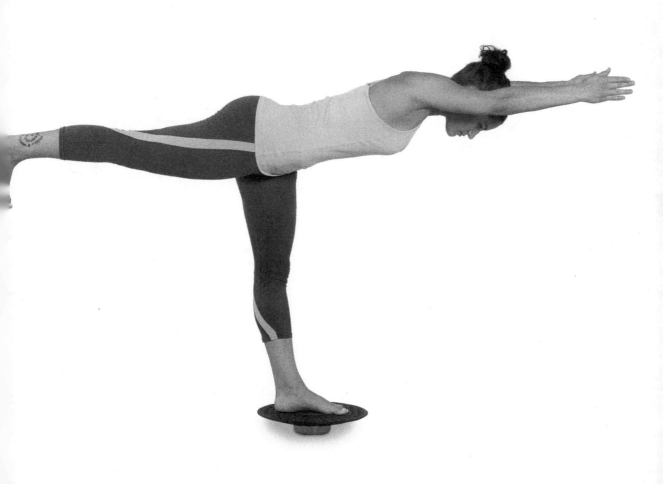

SEATED SERIES

SEATED ORIENTATION

TARGET: To acquaint the body with the balance board

Don't progress to any other exercises until you master this one!

1 Place the balance board on a firm surface such as a chair or bench. Sit on it and slowly find your balance point.

2–3 Once comfortable, slowly lean left and right, stopping along the way to catch your balance. Control the motion—don't allow momentum to move you.

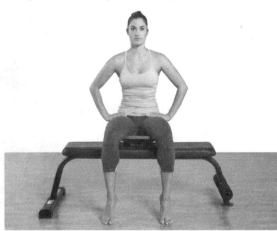

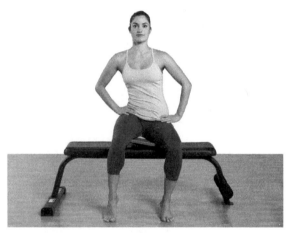

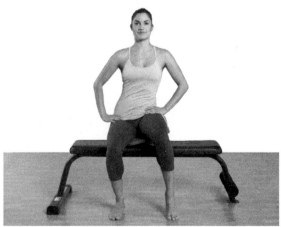

4 After you've competed a comfortable number of reps, try moving forward and backward several times.

Now try doing tailbone circles on the balance board in both directions.

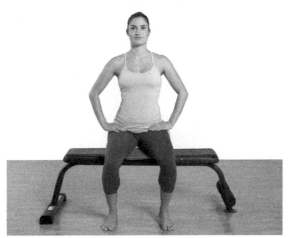

TARGET: Quadriceps, core

If you find this exercise too difficult, try it without weights.

1 Place the balance board on a firm surface such as a chair or bench. Strap an ankle weight to each ankle and sit with proper posture with your heels on the floor. Now slowly find your balance point.

2 Extend your right leg from the hip joint, keeping the leg straight and pointing your toes upward.

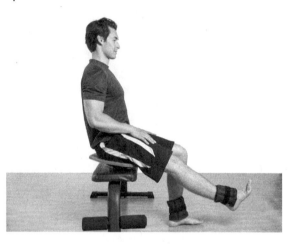

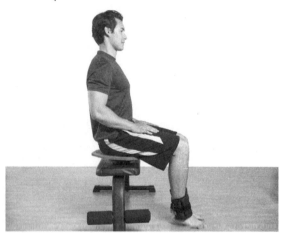

3 Lift your extended leg as high as is comfortable, but no higher than parallel with the floor. Hold for a moment.

Keeping the leg straight, slowly lower it to the floor. Alternate legs or repeat.

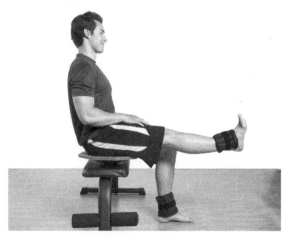

SEATED LEG EXTENSION

TARGET: Quadriceps, core

If you find this exercise too difficult, try it without weights.

1 Place the balance board on a firm surface such as a chair or bench. Strap an ankle weight to each ankle and sit with proper posture with your feet on or slightly off the floor and knees at a 90-degree angle. Now gently and slowly find your balance point.

2 Extend your right leg in front of you as high as is comfortable (but no higher than parallel with the floor).

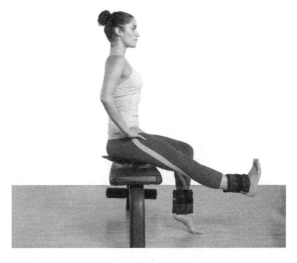

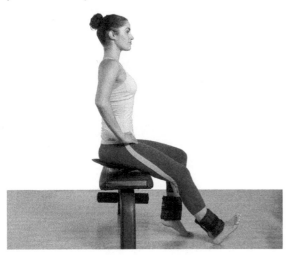

Slowly bend your knee. Alternate legs or repeat.

SEATED FRONTAL RAISE

TARGET: Shoulders, core

Only use a dumbbell if you can maintain balance while doing this exercise.

1 Place the balance board on a firm surface such as a chair or bench and sit on the board. Once you locate and maintain your balance point, grasp a comfortable dumbbell weight.

2 Slowly lift your arm forward to shoulder height.

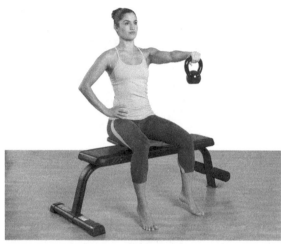

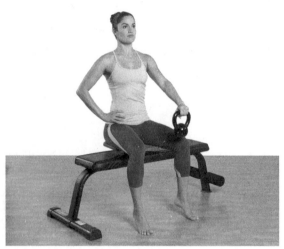

Slowly return your arm to start position.

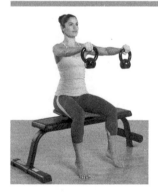

VARIATION: This can also be done with both arms at the same time.

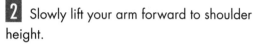

SEATED LATERAL RAISE

TARGET: Shoulders, core

Only use a dumbbell if you can maintain balance while doing this exercise.

1 Place the balance board on a firm surface such as a chair or bench and sit on the board. Once you locate and maintain your balance point, grasp a comfortable dumbbell weight.

2 Slowly lift your arm to the side to shoulder height.

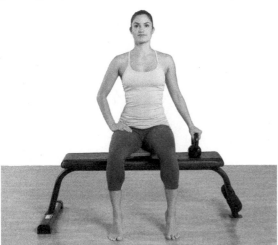

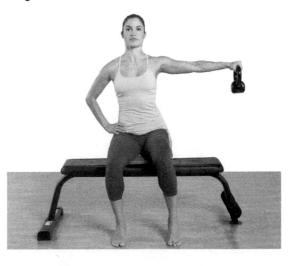

Slowly return your arm to start position.

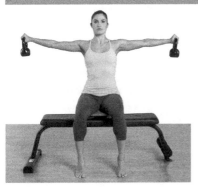

VARIATION: This can also be done with both arms at the same time.

SEATED SHOULDER PRESS

TARGET: Shoulders, core

Only use a dumbbell if you can maintain balance while doing this exercise.

1 Place the balance board on a firm surface such as a chair or bench and sit on the board. Once you locate and maintain your balance point, grasp a comfortable dumbbell weight.

2 Keeping your wrist in neutral position and your head and upper back in proper neutral position, slowly press your arm overhead. Pause when your arm is fully extended.

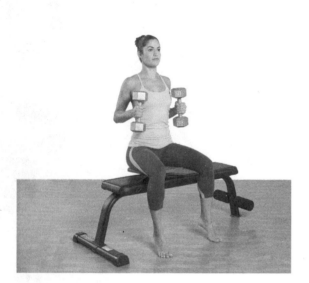

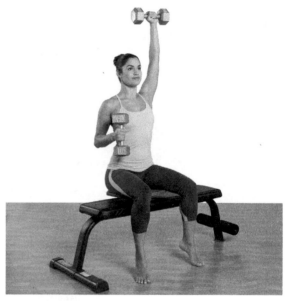

Slowly return to start position.

VARIATION: This can also be done with both arms at the same time.

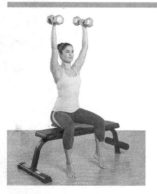

SEATED REVERSE FLY

TARGET: Upper back, core

1 Place the balance board on a firm surface such as a chair or bench. Sit on it and slowly find your balance point. While sitting upright with balanced posture, grasp an end of an exercise band in each hand at a location that provides the desired resistance and extend your arms in front of your chest.

2 While maintaining balance, extend your arms to the sides with control. Pause briefly.

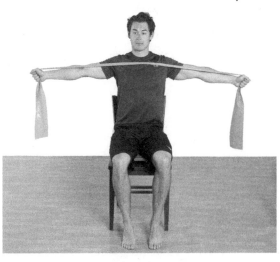

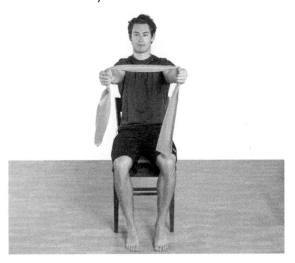

Return to start position.

TARGET: Triceps, core

1 Place the balance board on a firm surface such as a chair or bench. Sit on it and slowly find your balance point. While sitting upright with balanced posture, grasp an exercise band with both hands approximately shoulder-width apart and at chest height. Lift your elbows out to the sides, keeping your arms parallel to the floor.

2 Keeping your arms parallel to the floor, extend both arms to the sides.

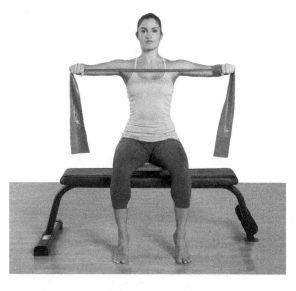

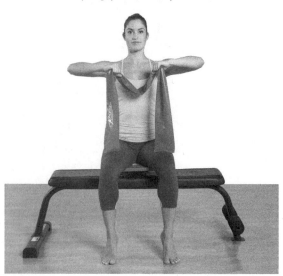

Slowly return to start position.

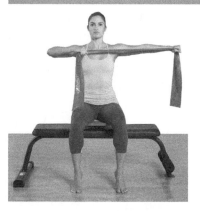

VARIATION: This can also be done with one arm at a time.

SEATED ROW

TARGET: Biceps, upper back, core

1 Place the balance board on the floor. Sit on it and slowly find your balance point. While sitting upright with balanced posture, wrap a band around both feet, extend your legs, then grasp the exercise band at a location that provides the desired resistance.

2 Keeping your wrist in neutral position and your head and upper back in proper neutral posture, slowly pull both ends of the band toward your waist.

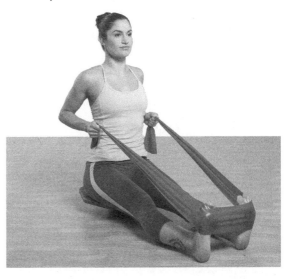

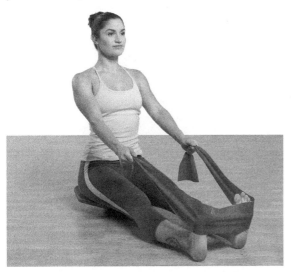

Slowly return to start position.

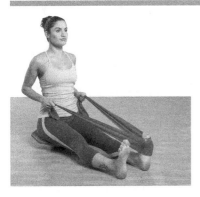

MODIFICATION: If balance is an issue, wrap the band around one foot only.

SEATED CHEST PRESS

TARGET: Chest, core

1 Place the balance board on a firm surface such as a chair or bench. Sit on it and slowly find your balance point. While sitting upright with balanced posture, place the band behind your mid-back, then grasp band at a location that provides the desired resistance near your shoulders.

2 Keeping your wrist in neutral position and your head and upper back in proper neutral posture, slowly press both ends of the band forward. Pause when both arms are extended in front.

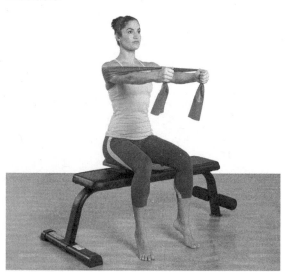

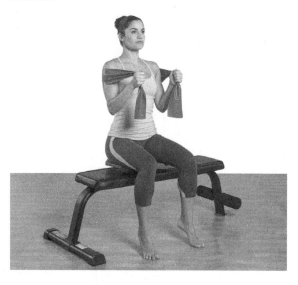

Slowly return to start position.

SEATED INCLINE CHEST PRESS

TARGET: Upper portion of chest, core

1 Place the balance board on a firm surface such as a chair or bench. Sit on it and slowly find your balance point. While sitting upright with balanced posture, place the band behind your mid-back, then grasp band at a location that provides the desired resistance near your shoulders.

2 Keeping your wrist in neutral position and your head and upper back in proper neutral posture, slowly press both ends of the band forward and upward at a 45-degree angle. Pause when both arms are extended in front.

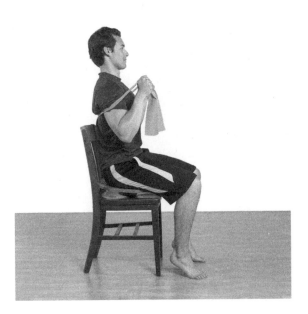

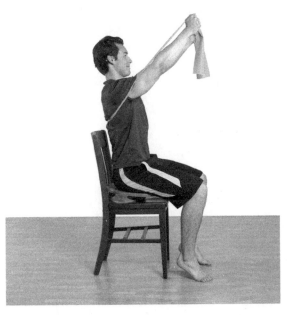

Slowly return to start position.

SEATED FLY

TARGET: Chest, core

1 Place the balance board on a firm surface such as a chair or bench. Sit on it and slowly find your balance point. While sitting upright with balanced posture, place the band behind your mid-back, then grasp the exercise band at a location that provides the desired resistance and extend your arms out to the sides.

2 While keeping tension in your arms, your wrist in neutral position and your head and upper back in proper neutral posture, slowly bring your hands toward each other in front of your chest.

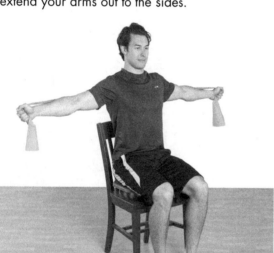

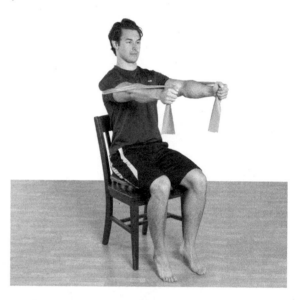

Slowly return to start position.

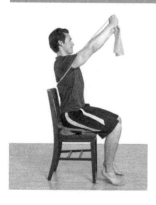

VARIATION: This can also be done with an incline by performing the exercise with your arms raised at a 45-degree angle.

TROMBONE SLIDE

TARGET: Triceps, anterior shoulder

1 Place the balance board on a firm surface such as a chair or bench. Sit on it and slowly find your balance point. While sitting upright with balanced posture, grasp an end of a band in each hand, holding your right hand near your chin and extending your left arm straight out in front of you.

2 Slowly bring your left arm back toward your chin and extend your right arm as if you were playing a trombone.

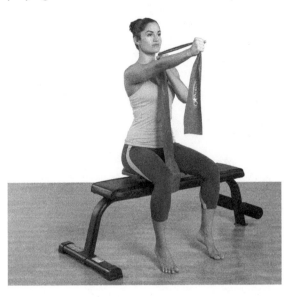

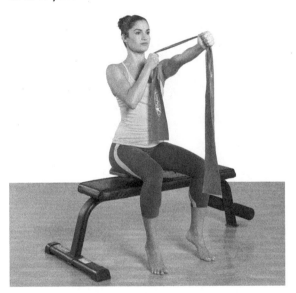

FLOOR SERIES

MAD CAT

TARGET: Lower back flexibility, wrist stability

1 While on your hands and knees, balance your hands on the balance board. Find and maintain your balance point.

2 Inhale and pull your bellybutton in to round your back.

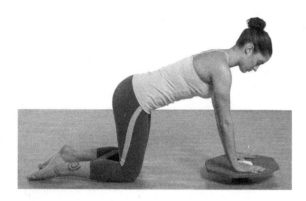

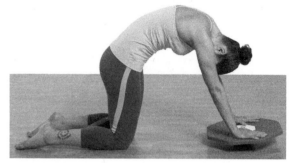

As you exhale, slowly relax your body to start position.

WRIST STRETCH

TARGET: Wrist flexibility

1 While on your hands and knees, place your hands with fingers pointing forward on the balance board. Find your balance point.

2–3 Slowly rock your hands forward and backward.

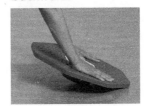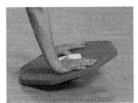

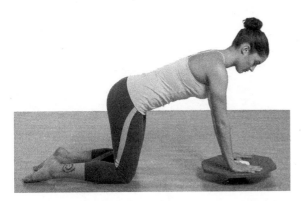

TARGET: Core and wrist stability

1 While on your hands and knees, balance your hands on the balance board. Find and maintain your balance point.

2 Once stable and stationary, raise one leg and hold.

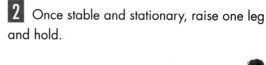

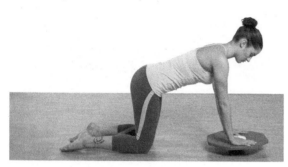

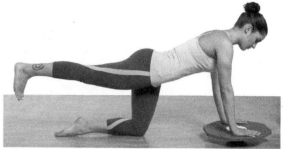

Lower it and repeat with the other leg.

PARTNER VARIATION: While doing the exercise, ask your partner to gently try to push you off balance as you maintain position.

WEIGHT VARIATION: Attach a weight to your ankle.

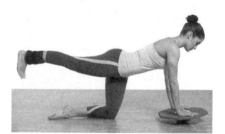

DONKEY KICK

TARGET: Core stability, gluteal toning

1 While on your hands and knees, balance your hands on the balance board. Find and maintain your balance point.

2–3 Draw your knee toward your chest, then kick the leg straight back and slightly upward.

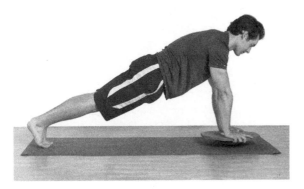

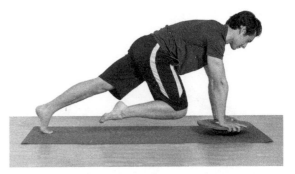

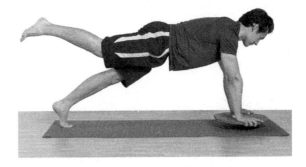

Repeat, and then switch sides. As you advance, you can alternate each leg while maintaining correct form.

MODIFICATION: This can also be done from your knees.

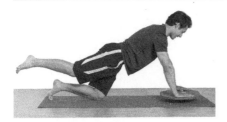

Exercises: Floor Series   **49**

PLANK TO PIKE

TARGET: Core, upper body

1 Place your feet on the balance board and assume a plank position with your hands on the floor, directly under your shoulders.

2 Raise your tailbone upward until you're an upside-down "V." You may need to walk your hands backward toward your feet.

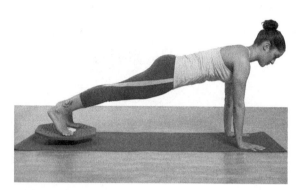 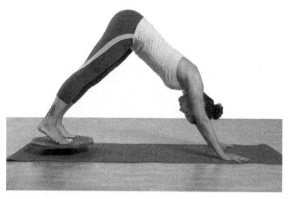

Lower to push-up position, then drop slightly below push-up position into a slight sag/arch position.

FOREARM PLANK

TARGET: Core

THE POSITION: Place your forearms on the floor with your elbows bent 90 degrees, then extend your legs behind you, placing your feet on the balance board. Make sure the board won't slip out from under you. Your body should form one plane from head to heels. Maintain a solid, straight position for a comfortable duration. Perfect form is critical! If you begin to sag or lift your tailbone, stop.

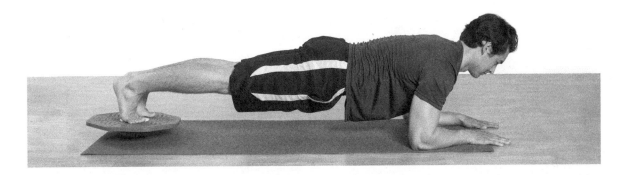

PLANK

TARGET: Core

THE POSITION: Place your hands on the balance board in a balanced position and then extend your legs behind you, placing your feet on the floor. Your legs can be spread apart to provide better balance but your body should form one straight line from head to heels. Hold correct form for as long as is comfortable. Perfect form is critical! If you begin to sag or lift your tailbone, stop.

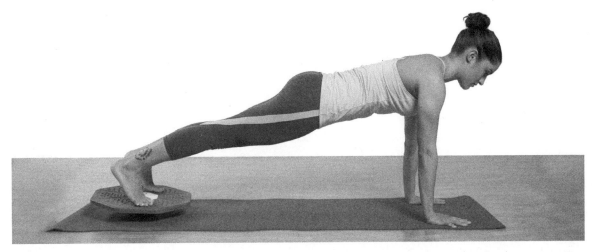

TRIPOD PLANK

TARGET: Core, upper body, glutes

1 Place your hands on the balance board and then extend your legs behind you, placing your feet on the floor.

2 Lift your right foot a comfortable distance off the ground.

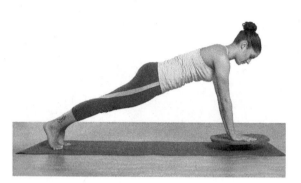

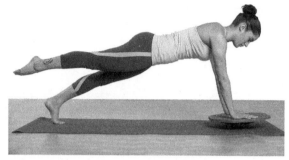

Place your right foot back on the ground and switch sides.

Continue alternating, stopping when perfect form is no longer maintained.

BIRD DOG

TARGET: Core, shoulder complex

1 Place your hands shoulder-width apart on the ground and extend your arms, extending your legs behind you so that your feet are balanced on the balance board.

2 Lift your right hand a comfortable distance off the ground.

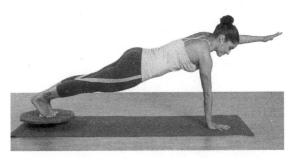

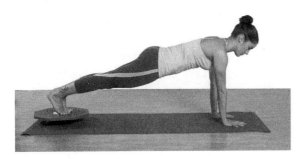

Place your right hand back on the ground and switch sides.

Continue alternating, stopping when perfect form is no longer maintained.

PUSH-UP

TARGET: Core, chest, shoulders, triceps, wrist stability

Once you start to sag in the middle or lift your butt, you have lost proper form—stop!

1 Assume a plank position with your hands in a secure position on the balance board.

2 Slowly lower your body to the floor, trying to keep your elbows close to your body. Only go as low as you feel comfortable and balanced.

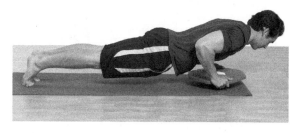

Return to start position.

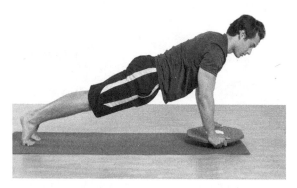

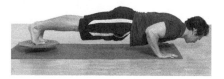

VARIATION: You can also perform this with your feet on the board.

DIAMOND PUSH-UP WITH BAND

TARGET: Core, chest, shoulders, triceps, wrist stability

Once you start to sag in the middle or lift your butt, you have lost proper form—stop!

1 Position a band around your upper back and under your arms. Place your hand in a diamond shape on the balance board and assume a plank position.

2 Slowly lower your body to the floor, trying to keep your elbows close to your body. Only go as low as you feel comfortable.

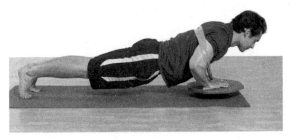

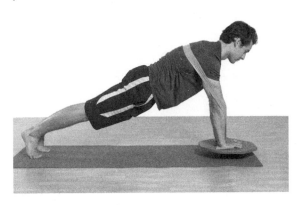

Extend your arms to start position.

SIDE PLANK

TARGET: Core, arms

THE POSITION: Assume a plank position with your hands on the floor and both feet on the balance board. Once you've found your balance point, slowly raise your left arm to the ceiling and rotate your torso toward the left, stacking your shoulders, hips, and feet atop each other.

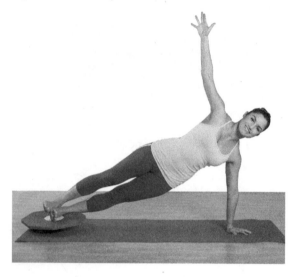

Return to start position and repeat on the other side.

ADVANCED VARIATION: For an even bigger challenge, try this with your hands on the balance board and your feet on the floor.

DIP

TARGET: Triceps

This requires a solid chair with arm rests.

1 With the balance board behind you, sit on the floor and place your hands on the balance board and feet on the floor, knees bent. Lift your butt a few inches off the ground.

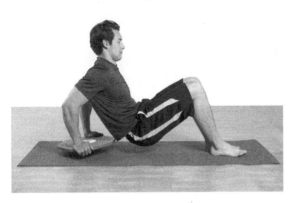

2 Straighten your arms, staying mindful of not rocking the balance board too much.

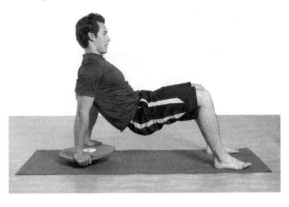

Bend your elbows and lower your rear end toward the ground.

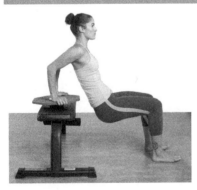

VARIATION: For an extra challenge, place the board on a higher surface.

PELVIC LIFT

TARGET: Core, glutes, ankle stability

1 Lie face up with your feet on the balance board and arms along your sides on the floor.

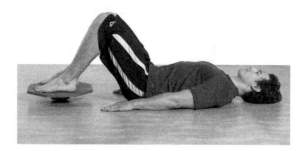

2 Squeezing your glutes, lift your tailbone upward a comfortable height.

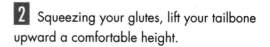
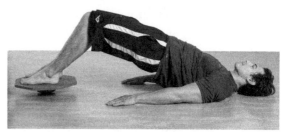

Lower yourself slowly.

WINDMILL

TARGET: Abdominals, shoulder flexibility

1 Lie face up on the floor with your feet on the balance board. Lift your tailbone upward and extend both arms toward the ceiling.

2 Keeping your tailbone elevated and maintaining core control, move one arm forward and the other backward.

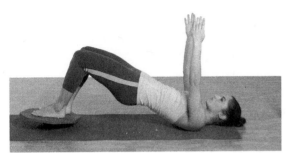

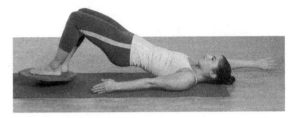

Continue alternating as long as you can avoid rocking.

CAN CAN KICK

TARGET: Abdominals, shoulder flexibility

For this exercise, it may be easier if the foot is placed closer to the middle of the balance board.

CAUTION: This exercise is known to cause hamstring cramps.

1 Lie face up on the floor with your feet on the balance board. Lift your tailbone upward and extend both arms toward the ceiling.

2 Keeping your tailbone elevated and maintaining core control, slowly extend one leg up to the ceiling.

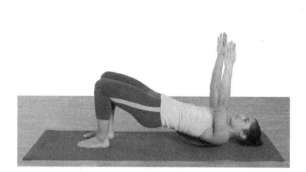
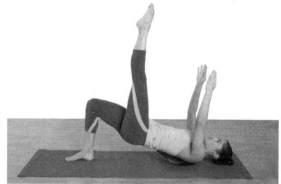

Lower the leg slowly and then extend the other leg. Continue alternating as long as you can avoid rocking.

PELVIC LIFT & CHEST PRESS

TARGET: Core, glutes, chest, arms

1 Lie face up on the floor with your feet on the balance board and arms along your sides on the floor. Hold a dumbbell in each hand with your hands in front of your shoulders.

2 Squeezing your glutes, lift your tailbone upward a comfortable height and press the dumbbells to the ceiling.

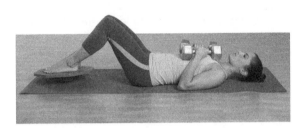

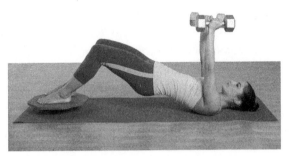

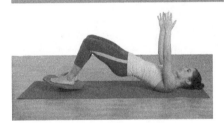

MODIFICATION: This can also be done without weights.

DEAD BUG

TARGET: Core, glutes, chest, arms

If you're lean and your balance board is hard, consider avoiding this exercise or place a towel on your board. Also, if your head is off the board, consider resting your head on a small pillow.

CAUTION: This exercise is known to cause hamstring cramps.

1 Lie on the floor face up and place the balance board under your shoulder blades. Bend your knees and place your feet on the floor. Squeezing your glutes, lift your tailbone upward a comfortable height. Once stable, lift both arms straight above your chest.

2 Move one arm forward and the other backward as you raise one leg to the ceiling. It's okay to experiment with which leg to raise.

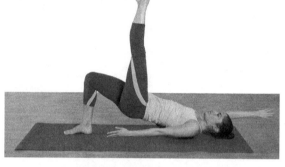

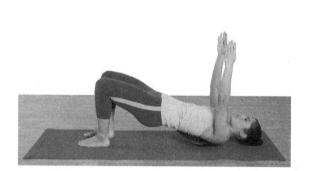

Continue alternating arms and legs.

BICYCLE

TARGET: Core

1 Place the balance board on the ground and sit on it. Lean back slightly, placing your hands on the ground for support or on the edges of the board. Once stable, lift your feet off the ground.

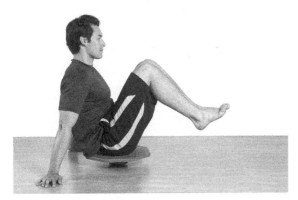

2 Bring one knee in to your chest as you extend your other leg forward and touch the heel to the ground.

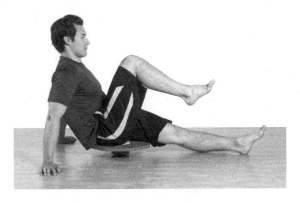

Continue alternating legs.

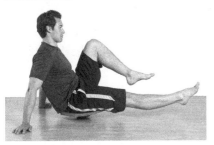

ADVANCED VARIATION: Try this without touching your heel on the ground.

CRUNCH

TARGET: Core

1 Place the balance board on the ground and sit on it. Lean back slightly, placing your hands on the ground for support or on the edges of the board. Once stable, lift your feet off the ground and pull both knees in toward your chest as far as is comfortable.

2 Now extend your legs forward, touching your heels to the ground.

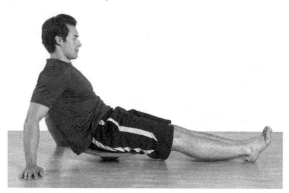

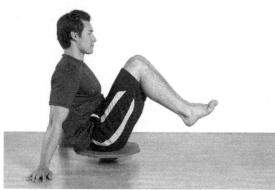

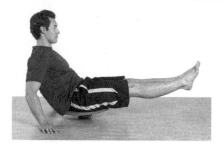

ADVANCED VARIATION: Try this without touching your heels on the ground.

CRAB KICK & DIP

TARGET: Core, glutes, triceps

Beginners should start with only one aspect of the exercise, such as just the leg kick or just the mini-dip.

1 With the balance board behind you, sit on the floor with your knees bent, both feet flat on the floor, and hands on the balance board. Once stable, straighten your arms and lift your rear end off the floor.

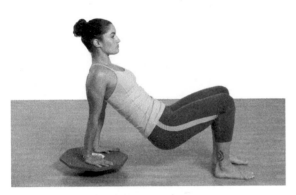

2–3 Keeping your knees close together, extend one leg forward and then the other.

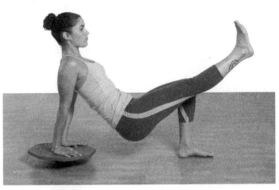

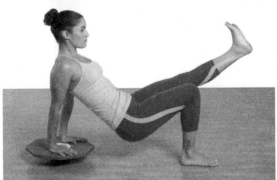

4 Lower your foot to the floor and bend your elbows to perform a mini-dip.

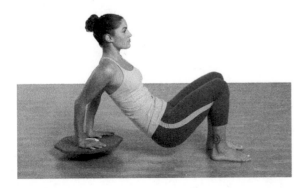

STANDING SERIES

STANDING STARTER

TARGET: Core, leg stamina

Stand near a chair for support.

CAUTION: Do not progress to other exercises until you're safe with this exercise.

1 Stand with your feet a comfortable distance apart and weight evenly supported on the balance board. Shift your weight until you find your balance point. Hold on to the back of the chair as needed. See how long you can maintain your balance. Your goal is to stand without holding on to the chair for 30 seconds or more.

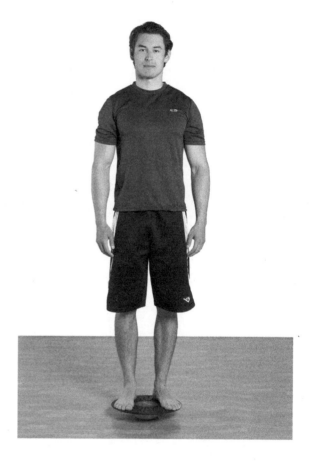

STANDING FORWARD LEAN

TARGET: Leg stamina

1 Stand with your feet a comfortable distance apart on the balance board and weight evenly supported. Shift your weight until you find your balance point.

2 Lean slightly forward as far as possible while maintaining balance. Try not to let the edges of the balance board touch the floor.

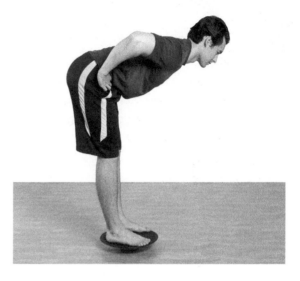

Return to start position.

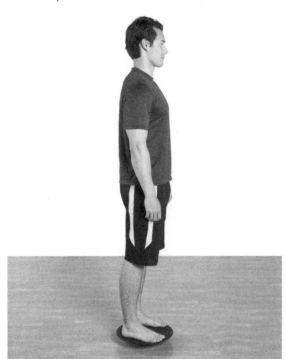

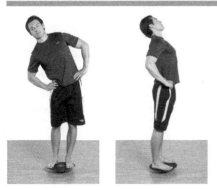

ADVANCED VARIATION: Try doing this move to both sides as well as back and forth without using any support.

CHAIR PUSH-UP

TARGET: Pectorals, core, triceps

You may place an exercise mat beneath the balance board and chair to prevent slippage. This can also be done against the wall.

CAUTION: Make sure the balance board won't slip out from under you while performing the push-up.

1 Stand on the balance board and place your hands shoulder-width apart on the back of a sturdy chair located a comfortable distance away from you. Your body will be approximately 45 degrees from the floor and your legs should be straight but not locked.

2 Keeping your torso in a straight line with your legs, lower your chest to the chair by bending your arms.

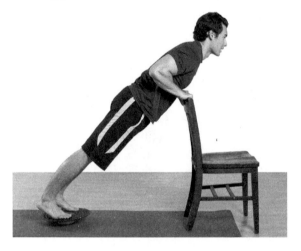

Press your body away until your arms are fully extended without being locked.

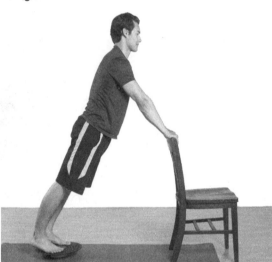

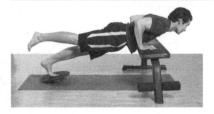

VARIATION: To increase resistance, use a sturdy surface, such as a coffee table or the seat of the chair, that's closer to the ground.

VARIATION: For an extra challenge, perform this with only one leg at a time on the board.

ROCK AROUND THE CLOCK

TARGET: Core, ankle flexibility

Stand near a chair or wall for support if necessary.

1 Stand on the balance board with your feet a comfortable distance apart and weight evenly supported.

2 By shifting your feet and body weight, move the board in a clockwise direction, then reverse direction.

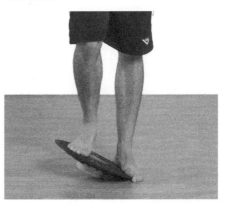

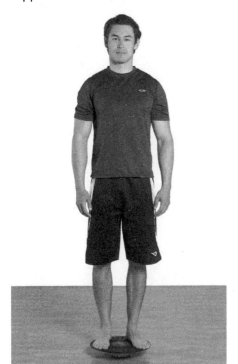

3 Rock forward and back.

4 Move side to side.

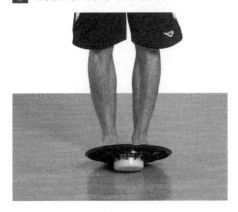

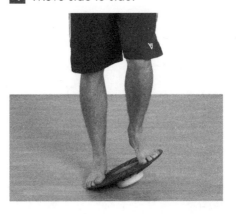

STANDING HULA

TARGET: Core, leg stamina

Stand near a chair or wall for support if necessary.

1 Stand on the balance board with your feet a comfortable distance apart and weight evenly supported.

2–3 Once you find your balance point, move only your hips in a clockwise manner.

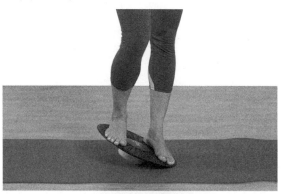

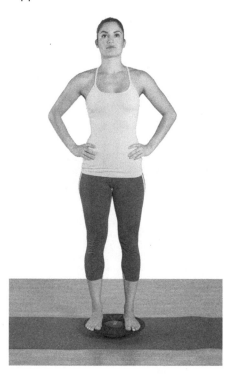

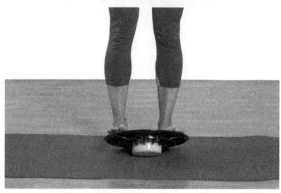

Reverse direction.

STANDING EMPIRE STATE BUILDING

TARGET: Core, leg and ankle stamina

Stand near a chair or wall for support if necessary.

1 Stand on the balance board with your feet a comfortable distance apart and weight evenly supported.

2–3 Looking up and down, see how long you can maintain your balance.

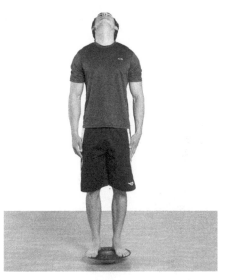

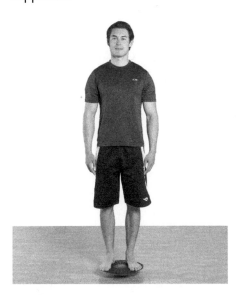

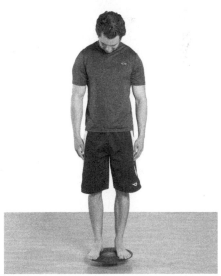

ADVANCED VARIATION: Once you master this move, try it with your eyes closed.

HALF SQUAT

TARGET: Core, leg stamina

Stand near a chair or wall for support if necessary.

1 Stand on the balance board with your feet a comfortable distance apart and weight evenly supported.

2 Lower yourself to a half-squat position. See how low you can go while still maintaining your balance.

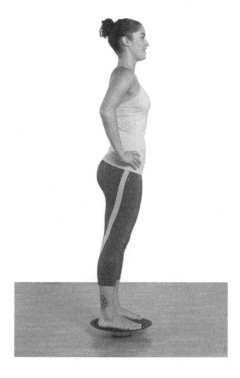

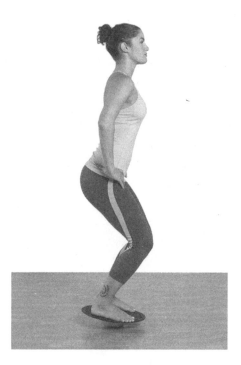

Return to start position.

ADVANCED VARIATION: Once you master this move, try it with your eyes closed.

FORWARD TOE TAP

TARGET: Static leg strength

Stand near a chair or wall for support if necessary.

1 Step onto the balance board with your left foot and place your right foot on the floor in front of the board.

2 Slowly bring your right foot to your left ankle.

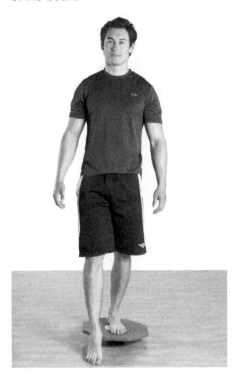

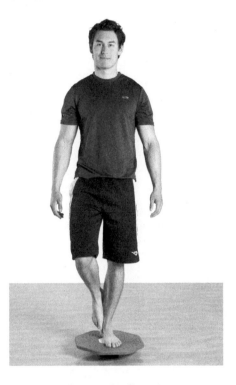

Return the foot to the floor.

Repeat, and then switch sides.

ADVANCED VARIATION: As you progress, just tap the toe to the ground.

LATERAL TOE TAP

TARGET: Static leg strength

Stand near a chair or wall for support if necessary.

1 Step onto the balance board with your right foot and place your left foot on the floor to the side of the board.

2 Slowly bring your left foot to your right ankle.

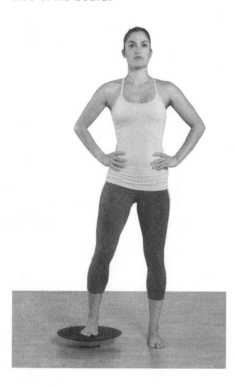

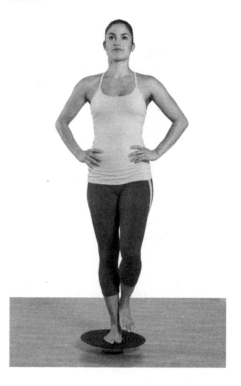

Return the foot to the floor.

Repeat, and then switch sides.

ADVANCED VARIATION: As you progress, just tap the toe to the ground.

FORWARD LUNGE

TARGET: Core, legs

Stand near a chair or wall for support if necessary.

1 Stand on the balance board with your feet a comfortable distance apart and weight evenly supported.

2 Once centered, step your right foot forward a comfortable distance, bending your knee up to 90 degrees as your foot lands.

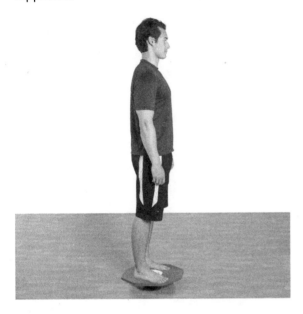

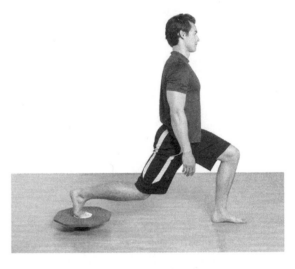

Return to start position.

Switch sides and continue alternating.

ADVANCED VARIATION: As you progress, try this with your eyes closed.

BACKWARD LUNGE

TARGET: Core, legs

Stand near a chair or wall for support if necessary.

1 Stand on the balance board with your feet a comfortable distance apart and weight evenly supported.

2 Once centered, step your left foot backward a comfortable distance, bending your knee up to 90 degrees as your foot lands.

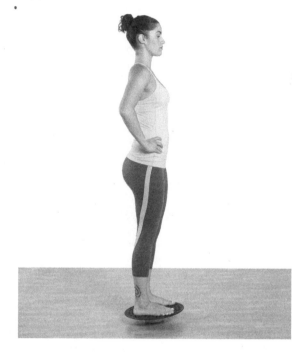

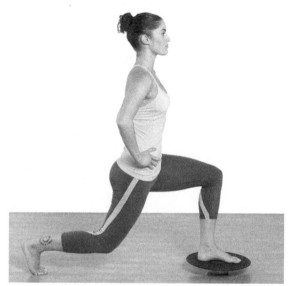

Return to start position. Switch sides and continue alternating.

ADVANCED VARIATION: As you progress, try this with your eyes closed.

SIDE STEP

TARGET: Core, legs

Stand near a chair or wall for support if necessary.

1 Stand on the balance board with your left foot on the balance board and your right foot on the floor to the side.

2 Once centered, step your right foot to the side a comfortable distance, bending your knee up to 90 degrees as your foot lands.

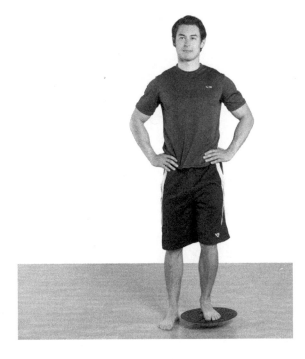 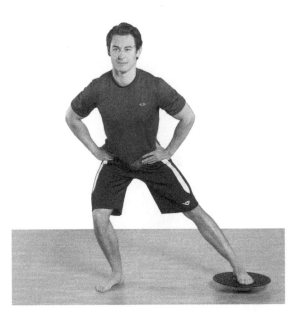

Return to start position.

Switch sides and continue alternating.

ADVANCED VARIATION: As you progress, try this with your eyes closed.

DYNAMIC SQUAT

TARGET: Core, leg stamina

Stand near a chair or wall for support if necessary.

1 Stand on the balance board with your feet a comfortable distance apart and weight evenly supported. Hold your arms either in front or to the side for balance.

2 Lower yourself up and down at a comfortable pace without losing your balance or rocking too much.

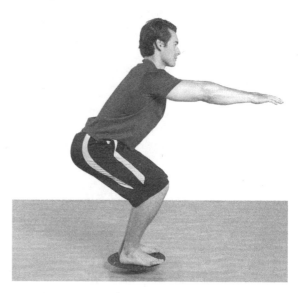

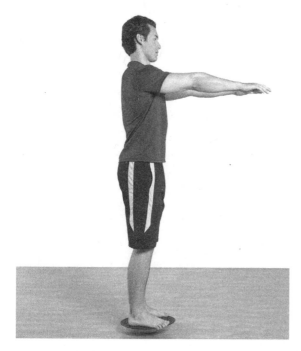

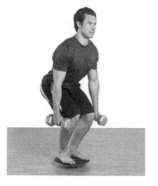

ADVANCED VARIATION: Once you master this move, try it with a kettlebell or dumbbell in each hand.

STANDING ARM SWING

TARGET: Static leg strength

1 Stand on the balance board with your feet a comfortable distance apart and weight evenly supported.

2 After finding your balance point, swing one arm forward and the other backward.

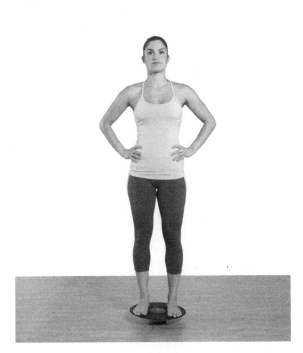

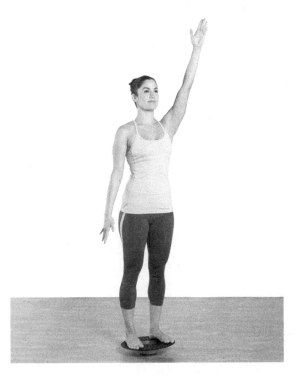

Continue alternating.

STANDING LATERAL ARM SWING

TARGET: Static leg strength

1 Stand on the balance board with your feet a comfortable distance apart and weight evenly supported.

2 After finding your balance point, keeping your arms straight, swing your arms across your chest and out to the sides.

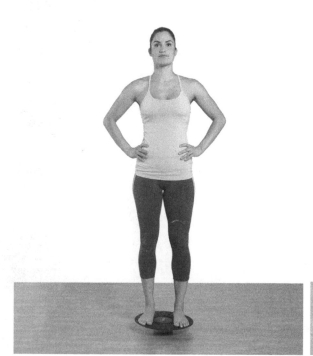
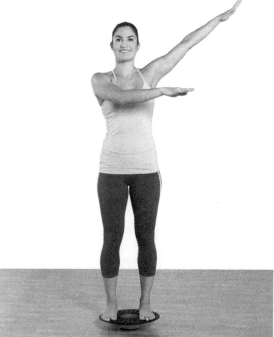

STANDING LATERAL RAISE

TARGET: Core, upper body, leg stamina

The goal of this advanced exercise is NOT how much you can lift but how many reps you can do while not losing balance.

1 Stand on the balance board with your feet a comfortable distance apart and weight evenly supported. Hold a dumbbell in each hand with your arms at your sides.

2 While maintaining your balance, lift your arms out to the sides, stopping at shoulder height.

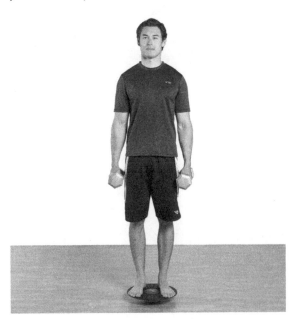

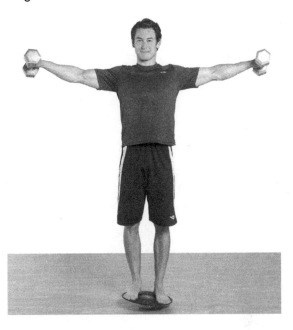

Return to start position.

STANDING FRONTAL RAISE

TARGET: Core, upper body, leg stamina

The goal of this advanced exercise is NOT how much you can lift but how many reps you can do while not losing balance.

1 Stand on the balance board with your feet a comfortable distance apart and weight evenly supported. Hold a dumbbell in each hand with your arms at your sides.

2 While maintaining your balance, lift your right arm forward, stopping at shoulder height.

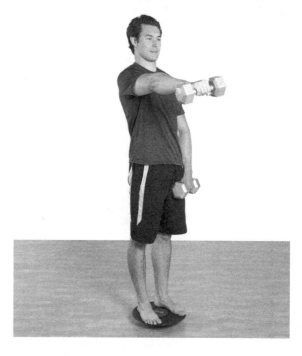

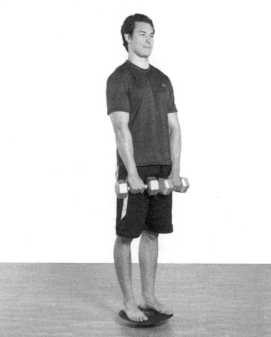

Return to start position and switch sides. Continue alternating.

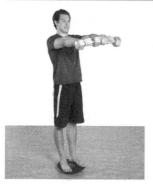

VARIATION: Simultaneously lift both arms forward.

STANDING ARM CURL

TARGET: Core, upper body, leg stamina

The goal of this advanced exercise is NOT how much you can lift but how many reps you can do while not losing balance.

1 Stand on the balance board with your feet a comfortable distance apart and weight evenly supported. Hold a dumbbell in each hand with your arms at your sides.

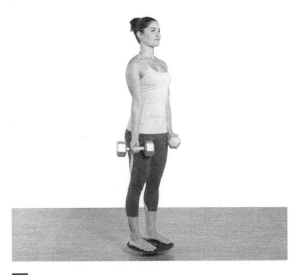

2 While maintaining your balance, curl the right dumbbell toward your shoulder.

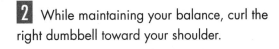

3 Return to start position and then repeat with your left arm.

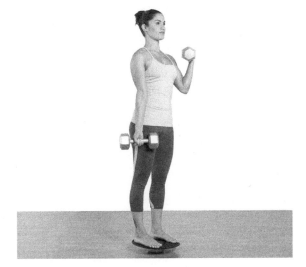

Continue alternating.

VARIATION: Simultaneously curl both arms.

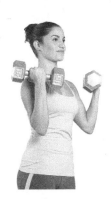

STANDING HORIZONTAL TRICEPS EXTENSION

TARGET: Core, upper body, leg stamina

The goal of this advanced exercise is performing reps while not losing balance.

1 Stand on the balance board with your feet a comfortable distance apart and weight evenly supported. With your elbows bent roughly 90 degrees and pointing out to the sides, grasp an exercise band with each hand at a location that provides the desired resistance.

2 While maintaining your balance and keeping your left hand in place, extend your right arm, pulling the band out to the right.

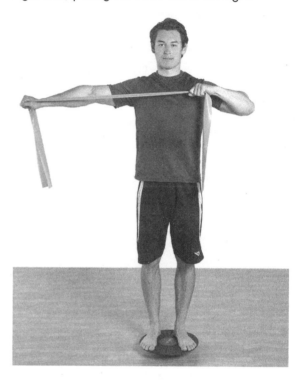

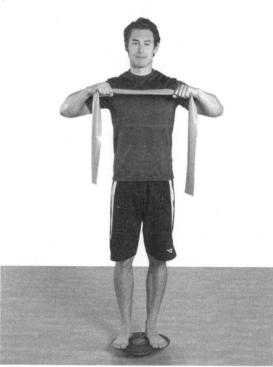

Return to start position and then perform with your left arm. Continue alternating.

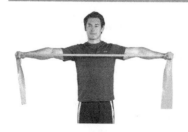

VARIATION: Simultaneously extend both arms.

STANDING HORIZONTAL FLY

TARGET: Core, upper body, leg stamina

The goal of this advanced exercise is performing reps while not losing balance.

1 Stand on the balance board with your feet a comfortable distance apart and weight evenly supported. With your arms straight out in front of you, grasp the exercise band with each hand at approximately shoulder distance.

2 Keeping your left arm in place and your right arm straight, take your right hand to the right side.

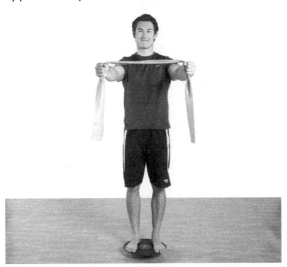

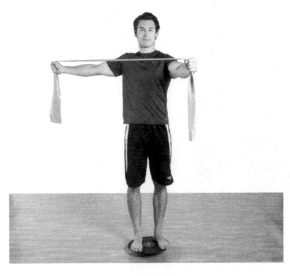

Return to start position and repeat with your left arm. Continue alternating.

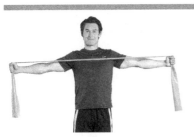

VARIATION: This can also be done with both arms at the same time.

STANDING ROW

TARGET: Core, upper body, leg stamina

1 Stand on the balance board with your feet a comfortable distance apart and weight evenly supported. Grasp a kettlebell, dumbbell or light barbell with both hands, arms hanging straight.

2 Keeping the weight close to your body, pull it up to chest height, allowing your elbows to go out to the sides.

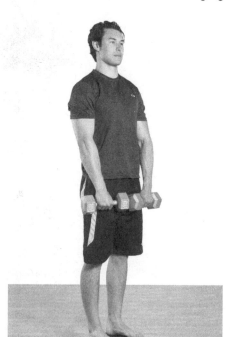

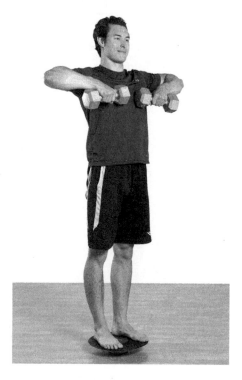

Lower the weight.

STANDING OVERHEAD PRESS

TARGET: Core, upper body, leg stamina

This is an advanced move.

CAUTION: Lifting a weight overhead can be dangerous. Do not do this exercise unless you're completely focused and have super balance.

1 Stand on the balance board with your feet a comfortable distance apart and weight evenly supported. Grasp a kettlebell, dumbbell or light barbell with both hands, arms hanging straight.

2–3 Curl the weight to your chest/shoulders and then press it overhead.

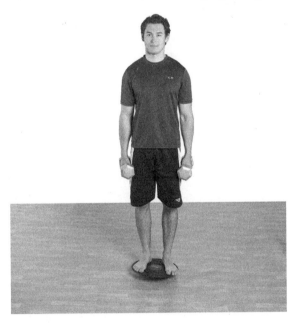

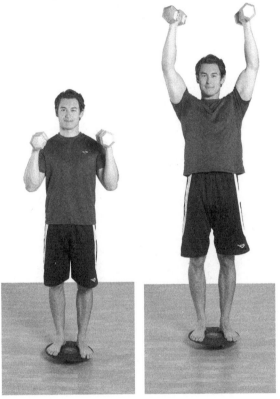

Lower the weight.

STORK STAND

TARGET: Core stability, leg endurance

This is an advanced move. Make sure the balance board won't slip!

1 Place one foot in the center of the balance board and the other foot on the floor a comfortable distance away. Find your balance point.

2 Once stable and stationary, raise the leg that's on the floor. You may move your arms to assist with balance. Aim to hold for up to 1 minute.

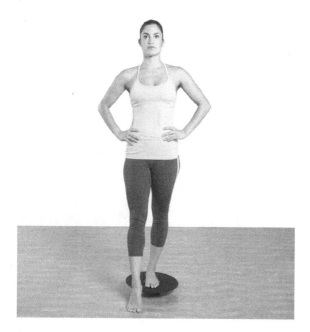

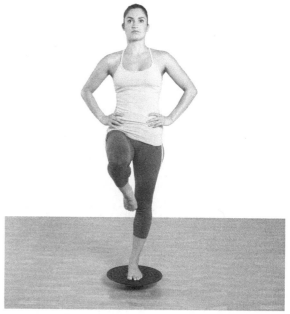

Switch sides.

SINGLE-LEG STAND WITH TORSO ROTATION

TARGET: Core, leg endurance

1 Place your left foot in the center of the balance board and the other foot on the floor a comfortable distance away. Find your balance point and bring your arms up to shoulder height as if hugging a large barrel. Maintain this arm position throughout the exercise.

2 Once steady, inhale and raise your left foot off the ground.

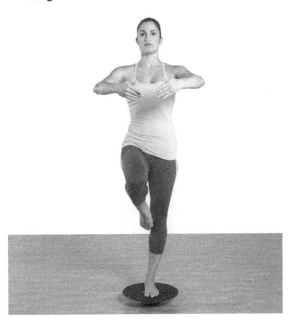

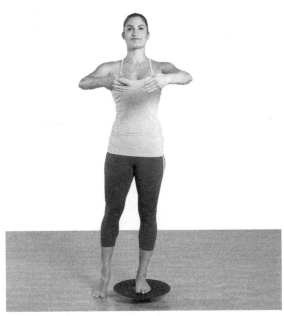

3 Exhale and rotate your upper body to the left, trying to keep your lower body pointing forward. Hold for a moment.

4 Inhale back to center.

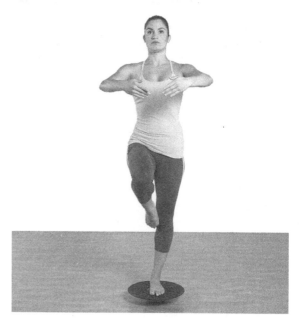

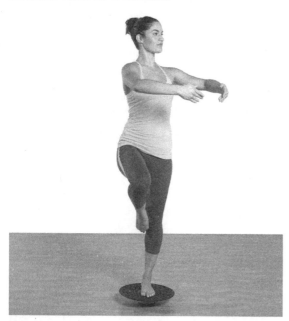

5 Exhale and rotate your upper body to the right. Hold for a moment.

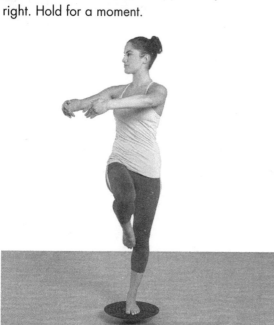

T STAND

TARGET: Core stability

This is an advanced move. Make sure the balance board won't slip!

1 Place one foot in the center of the balance board and the other foot on the floor a comfortable distance away. Find your balance point.

2 Once stable and stationary, raise the leg that's on the floor and slowly raise both arms to form a "T." Aim to hold for 30 seconds.

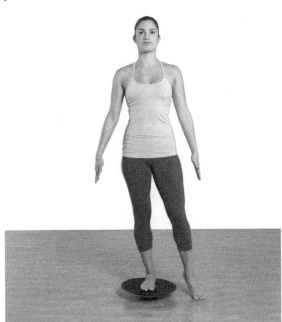

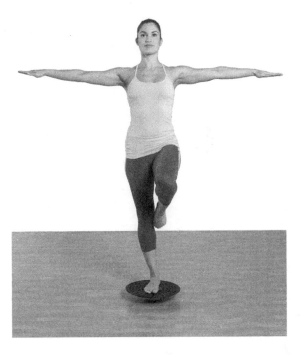

Switch sides.

OPPOSITE JACKS

TARGET: Core stability

This is an advanced move. Make sure the balance board won't slip out from under you!

1 Place your right foot in the center of the balance board and the other foot on the floor a comfortable distance away.

2 Once stable and stationary, raise your left leg and right arm out to the sides.

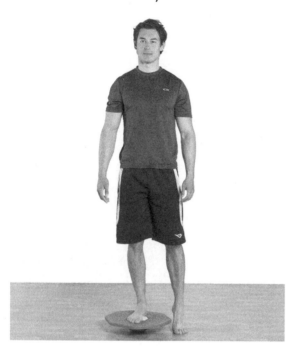

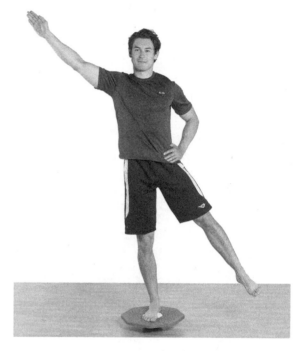

Repeat and then switch sides.

HALF JACKS

TARGET: Core stability

This is a VERY advanced move. Make sure the balance board won't slip out from under you!

1 Place your right foot in the center of the balance board and the other foot on the floor a comfortable distance away. Find your balance point.

2 Once stable and stationary, raise your left leg and left arm out to the side.

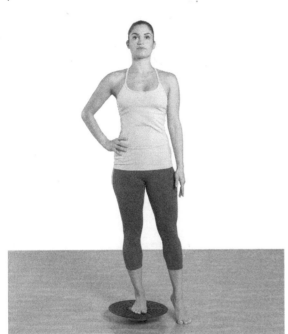

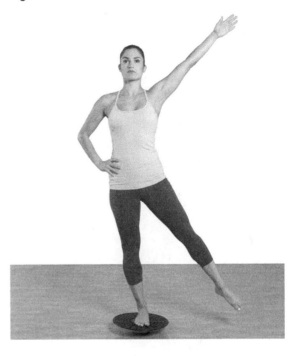

Repeat and then switch sides.

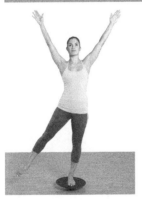

MODIFICATION: If balance is an issue, you may move both arms out to the sides.

TARGET: Core stability, hamstrings, leg endurance

This is an advanced move that can also be performed with an ankle weight. Make sure the balance board won't slip out from under you!

1 Place your right foot in the center of the balance board and the other foot on the floor behind you. Find your balance point. Take your arms out to the sides if necessary.

2 Once steady, bend your left knee, bringing your heel toward your buttock as close as possible.

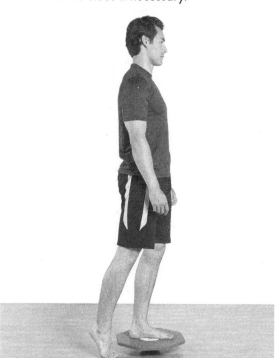

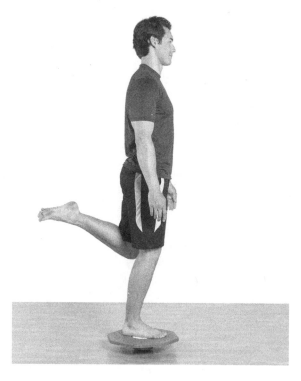

Lower your leg without placing your foot on the floor, if possible. Repeat and then switch sides.

SINGLE-LEG EXTENSION

TARGET: Core stability, leg endurance

This is an advanced move.

1 Place your left foot in the center of the balance board and the other foot on the floor in front of you. Find your balance point. Take your arms out to the sides if necessary.

2 Once steady, slowly kick your left leg forward as high as is comfortable.

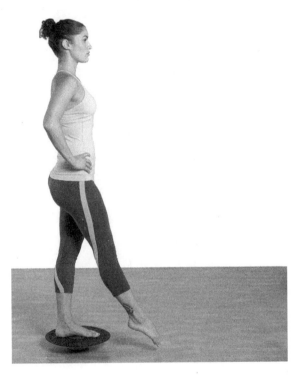

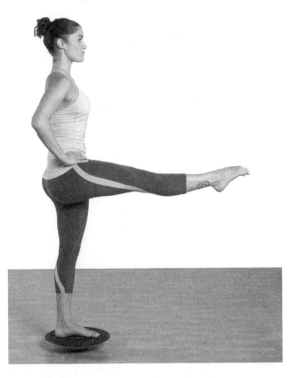

Continuing kicking, if possible, without placing your left foot on the floor.

Switch sides.

TARGET: Core stability, leg endurance

This is an advanced move.

1 Place your left foot in the center of the balance board and the other foot on the floor behind you. Find your balance point. Take your arms out to the sides if necessary.

2 Once steady, lift your left leg off the floor and slowly move it backward a comfortable distance. Keep your core engaged—staying balanced is the key, not distance.

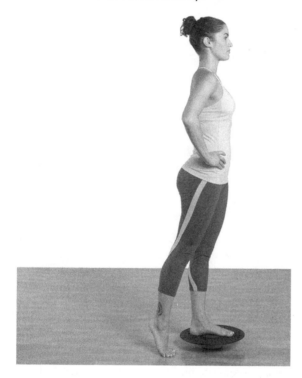

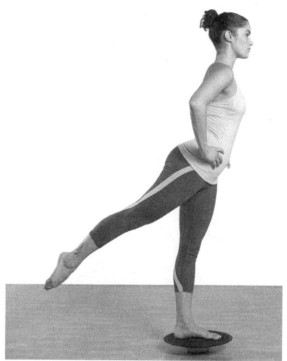

Return to start position. Repeat and switch sides.

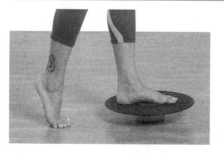

MODIFICATION: If you need extra support, you can slide your foot backward, keeping your toes on the floor.

LATERAL SINGLE-LEG RAISE

TARGET: Core stability, leg stamina

This is an advanced move.

1 Place your left foot in the center of the balance board and the other foot on the floor to the side. Find your balance point. Take your arms out to the sides if necessary.

2 Once steady, slide your left foot along the floor to the side. Keep your core engaged—staying balanced is the key, not distance.

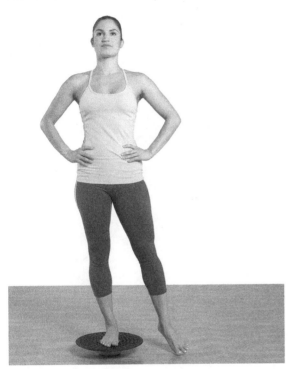

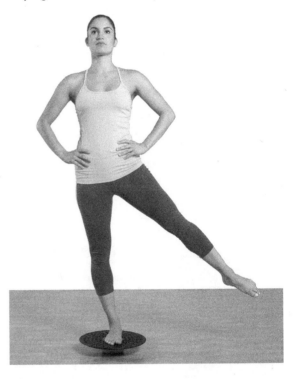

Return to start position. Repeat and switch sides.

ADVANCED VARIATION: Don't let your toes touch the ground.

SCALES

TARGET: Core stability, leg stamina

This is an advanced move.

1 Place your left foot in the center of the balance board and the other foot on the floor behind you. Find your balance point. Place your hands on your hips.

2 Once steady, lean forward from your hips until your back foot lifts off the floor. Keeping your body nice and straight, continue bending at the hip until you form a line from head to heel.

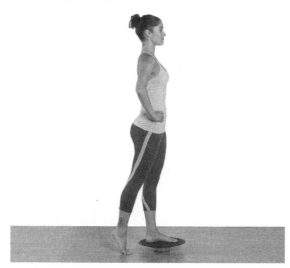

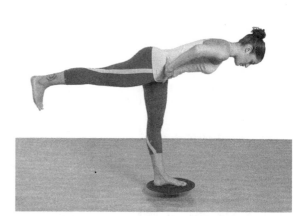

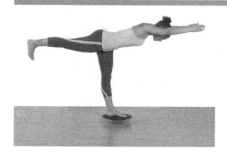

VARIATION: For an extra challenge, reach your arms forward so that your head is between your arms.

STRETCHES

CALF STRETCH

TARGET: Calf

THE POSITION: Stand tall with good posture, place your left foot on the center of the balance board, and then take your right leg as far back as you can, keeping your heel down. Bending your left knee slightly for balance and keeping your right heel down, press your hips forward and gently lean back until the desired stretch is felt in the calf, hip flexor and low back area. Hold this stretch for a comfortable moment. Switch sides.

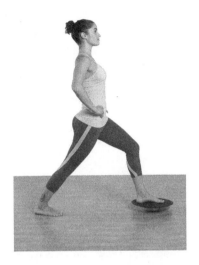

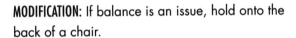

MODIFICATION: If balance is an issue, hold onto the back of a chair.

QUADRICEPS STRETCH

TARGET: Quadriceps

This is an advanced stretch. Please use caution.

THE POSITION: Stand with your feet a comfortable distance apart and weight evenly supported on the balance board. Once balanced, slowly bring your right heel to your right buttock, holding your foot with your right hand. Hold this stretch for a comfortable moment. Switch sides.

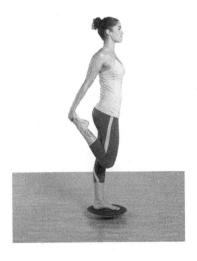

MODIFICATION: If balance is an issue, hold onto the back of a chair.

HAMSTRING STRETCH

TARGET: Hamstrings

This is an advanced stretch. Do not do this exercise if you get light-headed bending over.

THE POSITION: Stand with your feet a comfortable distance apart and weight evenly supported on the balance board. Once balanced, bend from the waist and attempt to touch the floor, straightening your legs if possible. Place your hands on your thighs for support if necessary.

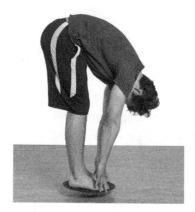

MODIFICATION: If balance is an issue, hold onto the back of a chair.

DOUBLE WOOD CHOP

TARGET: Upper body, chest, shoulders

This is an advanced move since no support is allowed.

1–2 Stand on the balance board with your feet a comfortable distance apart and weight evenly supported. Position your hands in front of your body and interlace your fingers. Inhale deeply through your nose and slowly raise both arms in front of you to a comfortable height. Hold 1–2 seconds.

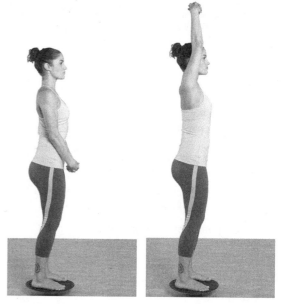

Exhale and slowly lower your arms to start position.

SOUP CAN POUR

TARGET: Shoulders

1 Stand on the balance board with your feet a comfortable distance apart and weight evenly supported. Shift your weight until you find your balance and then place your arms at your side and your palms facing back.

2 Inhale deeply through your nose and bring both arms slightly forward as you raise them out to the sides, keeping your palms facing back. Raise your arms no higher than shoulder level.

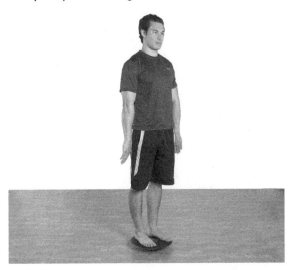

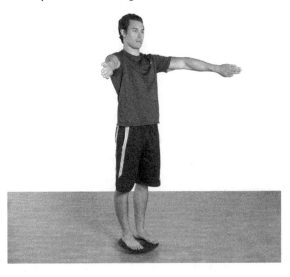

Exhale as you lower your arms.

HANDS BEHIND THE BACK

TARGET: Shoulders, chest

This is an advanced move since no support is allowed.

1–2 Stand on the balance board with your feet a comfortable distance apart and weight evenly supported. Attempt to interlace your fingers behind your back and then straighten your arms behind you. Focus on squeezing your shoulder blades together. Hold this position for as long as is comfortable.

MODIFICATION: If you can't reach behind you, you can hold the ends of a strap in each hand behind your bottom, or hold a bar.

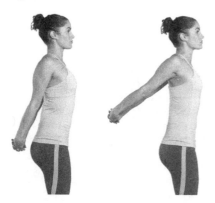

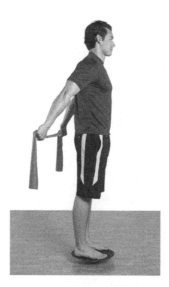

PEC STRETCH

TARGET: Shoulders, chest

This is an advanced move since no support is allowed.

THE POSITION: Stand on the balance board with your feet a comfortable distance apart and weight evenly supported. Place your hands behind your head. Gently move your elbows back and try to bring your shoulder blades together. Focus on opening up your chest and tightening your upper back muscles. Only go as far back as is comfortable and hold for a moment. Don't strain; breathe comfortably.

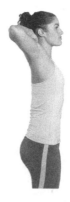

THE ZIPPER

TARGET: Shoulders

This is an advanced move since no support is allowed.

1 Stand on the balance board with your feet a comfortable distance apart and weight evenly supported. Place your right hand on your upper back behind your head. Take your left arm behind your back and grab your right fingertips with your left fingertips. Hold the position for a comfortable moment. Switch sides and repeat.

MODIFICATION: If you can't reach, hold an end of a strap in your upper hand, letting your lower hand grab the other end. Raise your right hand up as high as possible to lift your lower hand, staying in your pain-free zone, then pull down with your lower hand to bring down your higher hand.

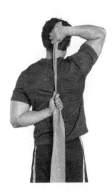

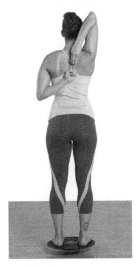

ELBOW TOUCH

TARGET: Chest, upper back

This is an advanced move since no support is allowed.

1 Stand on the balance board with your feet a comfortable distance apart and weight evenly supported. Place your right hand on your right shoulder and your left hand on your left shoulder.

2 Slowly attempt to bring your elbows together while maintaining good balance. Hold this stretch for a comfortable moment.

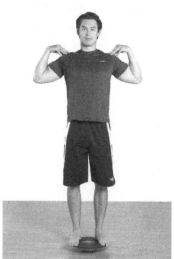

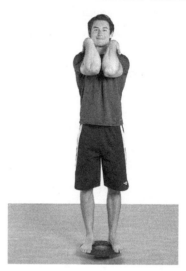

TARGET: Shoulder mobility

1 Stand on the balance board with your feet a comfortable distance apart and weight evenly supported. Place your right hand on your right shoulder and your left hand on your left shoulder.

2 Slowly reach as high as you can with your right hand while maintaining good balance.

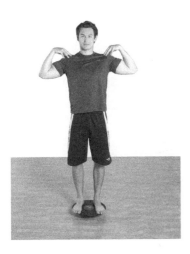

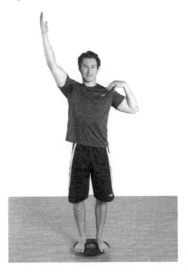

Return to start position and alternate sides.

CHOKER

TARGET: Shoulder flexibility

THE POSITION: Stand on the balance board with your feet a comfortable distance apart and weight evenly supported. Place your right hand on your left shoulder and then place your left hand on your right elbow. Gently press your right biceps toward your throat and hold for a moment. Release and switch sides.

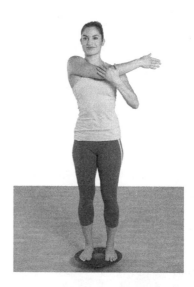

NECK STRETCH

TARGET: Neck

CAUTION: Avoid this if you have neck issues.

THE POSITION: Stand on the balance board with your feet a comfortable distance apart and weight evenly supported. Place your right hand on the left side of your head. While maintaining good balance, gently pull your head toward your left shoulder. Return to start position and switch sides.

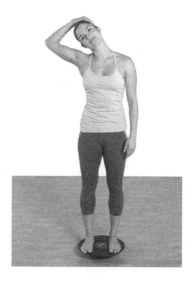

THE WATCHER

TARGET: Neck mobility

1–2 Stand on the balance board with your feet a comfortable distance apart and weight evenly supported. Slowly look left and then right while maintaining your balance.

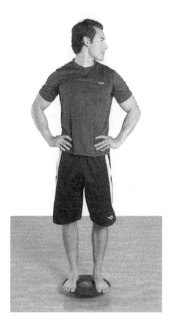
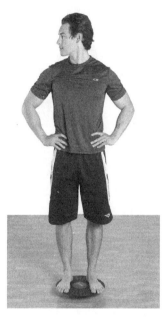

TWISTER

TARGET: Dynamic balance

1 Holding onto the back of a chair, stand on the balance board with your feet a comfortable distance apart and weight evenly supported posture.

2–3 Slowly twist your body left and right.

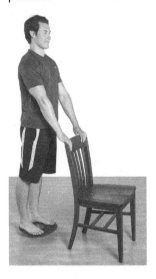

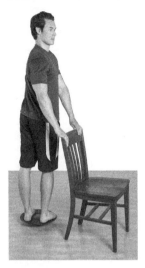 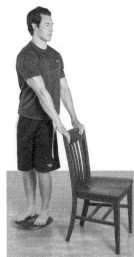

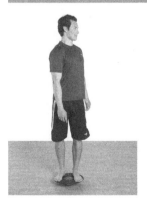

ADVANCED VARIATION: You can try this without support—just make sure the area around you is safe in case you fall. Some people can rotate all the way around.

KNEE ROLL

TARGET: Torso, hips

CAUTION: If you have low back problems, avoid this move.

1 Lie on a mat with your knees bent and your feet flat on the floor. Place your arms straight out to your sides in a "T" position.

2 While inhaling through your nose, allow your knees to drop gently to the right without discomfort. Exhale and hold this position for a comfortable moment.

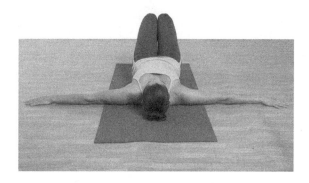

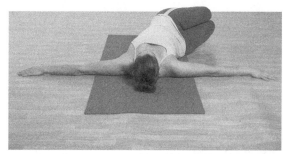

3 Inhale and bring your knees back to center, then gently drop them to your left. Exhale and hold this position for a comfortable moment.

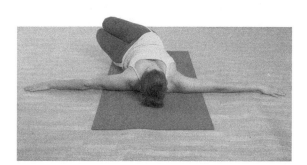

CROSS-LEG DROP

TARGET: Torso, piriformis

CAUTION: Be careful if you have low back problems.

1 Lie on a mat with your knees bent and your feet flat on the floor.

2 While focusing on your breathing, place your left knee on top of your right knee.

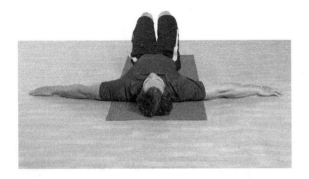

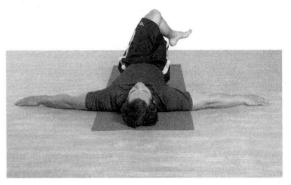

3 Slowly allow your left knee to gently fall toward the right side. Stop when you feel tightness. Hold this position for a comfortable moment. The stretch should be felt near the rear pocket area of the right leg. Focus on the stretch, not on how close you can bring your knees to the floor.

Switch sides and repeat.

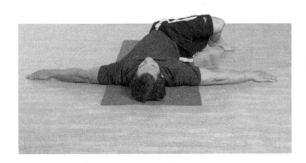

SINGLE KNEE TO CHEST

TARGET: Low back, gluteus maximus

1 Lie on a mat and, if needed, place a pillow under your head. Bend your knees and place both feet flat on the floor.

2 Gently grab behind the back of your left leg and bring your knee toward your chest. Hold this stretch for a comfortable moment.

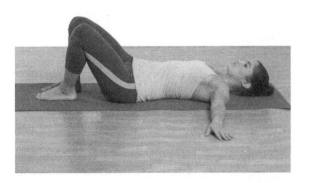

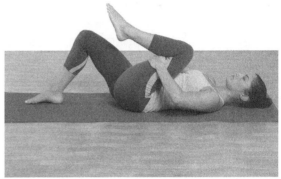

Release the knee, switch sides and repeat.

MODIFICATION: If you can't reach your leg, loop a strap behind the back of your right leg and hold an end of the strap in each hand.

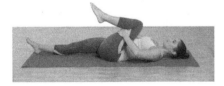

VARIATION: Extend one leg straight on the floor and bring one knee to your chest.

ROLL INTO A BALL

TARGET: Low back, gluteus maximus, torso

You might know this as "Child's Pose" if you do yoga.

CAUTION: Do not do this stretch if you have knee problems.

1 Place your hands and knees on the floor. Inhale through your nose. While exhaling deeply through your mouth, slowly allow your bottom to drop toward your heels. If you feel discomfort, you may place a pillow between your heels and bottom. Place your forehead on the floor or a pillow and position your arms alongside your body. Hold this position for a comfortable moment, enjoying the sensation of the stretch up and down your back.

VARIATION: If you can find a friend to rub up and down your back while doing this stretch, it will enhance the stretch.

ADVANCED: Stretch your arms out straight in front of you.

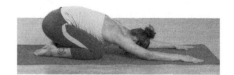

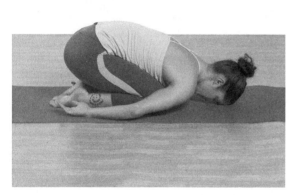

INDEX

ACKNOWLEDGMENTS

A special thanks goes out to Kelly Reed for her vision, along with the behind-the-scenes team at Ulysses Press. A special shout out goes to Lily Chou for making sense of my writing, as well as the rest of the editorial team, Claire Chun.

Another thought of appreciation goes to Rapt Productions and the models Nadia Brunner-Velasquez and Christopher Wells.

Last but not least, thank you to my son Chris for his critical suggestions on content of the book, and Margaret, my wife, for putting me out on a limb for the balance shot. Let's not leave out my other son Kevin for reminding me to laugh.

OTHER KARL KNOPF BOOKS

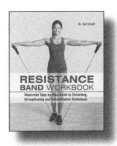

Resistance Band Workbook
$14.95
The ultimate tool for targeting, developing and healing every major muscle group, the resistance band is inexpensive, effective and portable. This book provides the most helpful workouts for noticeable results.

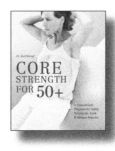

Core Strength for 50+
$15.95
Core Strength for 50+ provides the exercise and workout schedules that show anyone how to build and maintain strong muscles in the abs, obliques, lower back, butt and hips.

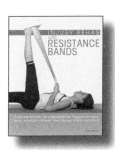

Injury Rehab with Resistance Bands
$15.95
Whether trying to reduce pain, transform troublesome muscles, or get back in the game, this handbook offers the most comprehensive rehab plan for any injury.

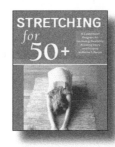

Stretching for 50+
$14.95
Based on the belief that individuals over 50 can do most of the same things as 20- and 30-year-olds, this book shows how to maintain and improve flexibility by incorporating stretching into one's life.

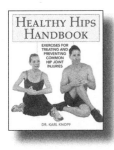

Healthy Hips Handbook
$14.95
Healthy Hips Handbook is designed to help prevent hip problems for some and, for those with existing hip problems, provide post-rehabilitation exercises.

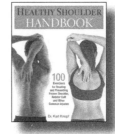

Healthy Shoulder Handbook
$15.95
Includes an overview of shoulder anatomy so anyone can use this friendly manual to strengthen an injured shoulder, identify the onset of a shoulder problem or better understand injury prevention.

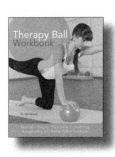

Therapy Ball Workbook
$14.95
Designed for more than just rehab, this book provides a complete program for using therapy balls to maintain a flexible, strong body and prevent future injury.

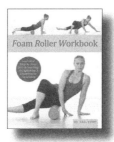

Foam Roller Workbook
$14.95
Details a comprehensive program for using the foam roller to recover from injury, reverse everyday pain and stay healthy in the future.

To order these books call 800-377-2542 or 510-601-8301, fax 510-601-8307, e-mail ulysses@ulyssespress.com, or write to Ulysses Press, P.O. Box 3440, Berkeley, CA 94703. All retail orders are shipped free of charge. California residents must include sales tax. Allow two to three weeks for delivery.

ABOUT THE AUTHOR

DR. KARL KNOPF, or Dr. Karl, as his students used to call him, has been involved in the health and fitness of older adults and the disabled for over 40 years. During this time he has worked in almost every aspect of the industry, from personal training and therapy to consultation.

While at Foothill College, Karl was the coordinator of the Adaptive Fitness Technician Program and Life Long Learning Institute. He taught disabled students and undergraduates about corrective exercise. In addition to teaching, Karl developed the "Fitness Educators of Older Adults Association" to guide trainers of older adults. Currently Karl is a director at the International Sports Science Association is on the advisor board of PBS's *Sit and Be Fit* show.

In his spare time he has spoken at conferences, authored many articles, and written numerous books on topics ranging from water workouts to fitness therapy. He was a frequent guest on both radio and print media on issues pertaining to senior fitness and the disabled.

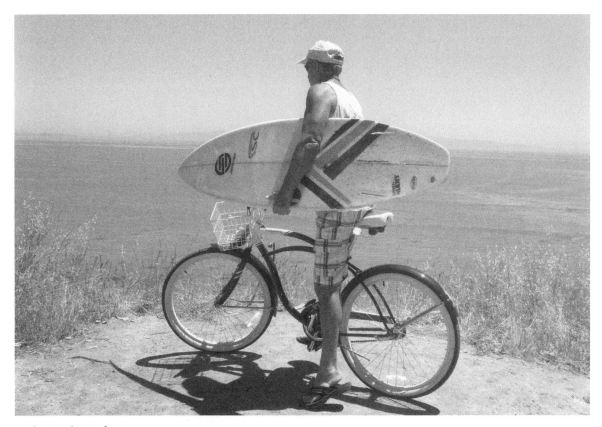

Author Karl Knopf enjoying retirement.